READERS' COMMENTS ABOUT
AN INTERNET GUIDE FOR THE HEALTH PROFESSIONAL, 2ND EI
and
A POCKET GUIDE TO THE MEDICAL INTERNET

The Medical Resource List is superb. I found I was able to utilise it right away for reference questions...This up-to-date book is written in a way that cuts through the theory, and generally gets straight to what the reader wants to know...This is a comprehensive, well-done book which will be a useful tool for getting your health professional started with the Internet and excited about its possibilities and uses...All in all, this book covers a huge amount of information in a simple, easy-to-read manner.

Sue Kurucz, Journal of Canadian Health Libraries Association, Spring 1996

My Russian translation of *A Pocket Guide to the Medical Internet* is used by all our 25 Regional Scientific Medical Libraries and it is very popular among our customers, especially health professionals from Research Institutes.

Victor Kalmykov, Head of Automation Department,
State Scientific Medical Library (Ukraine)

In my experience as a medical book vendor, I have never seen a book so widely and enthusiastically embraced.

Nora N. Hogan, UC Davis Medical Bookstore (California)

Your book is a teaching goldmine!

RN Instructor, University of Hawaii

Thank you for making your book available to all healthcare professionals.

Ronald T. Kneusel, Research Asst., Internal Medicine,
Medical College of Wisconsin

We are overjoyed to receive a copy of your second edition in our hospital.

Maria de Fatima de Castro Costa, MD, Neurology (Brazil)

The format and content are attractive, user-friendly and very useful. Thanks so much for your generous contribution to understanding the Internet.

Janet Conboy, Missouri Dept. of Mental Health

Hopefully, you will continue to provide your expert guidance to the development of California's public health information system.

Gwendolyn Doebbert, Asst. Chief for Health Information, California Dept. of Health Services

I was so excited to see your book. You are doing a great service; this is what we need to help pull health professionals into the current technology.

Frances A. McHolm, RN, MSN, Asst. Professor of Nursing, Malone College (Ohio)

If only I had had this book six months ago when I started learning to search the new medical resources for myself...As much as doctors need this resource, the 20 million of us out here in the U.S. who have rare/chronic diseases need it even more...I can't wait to see what you have, and I am hoping to learn a lot from reading the book.

Christina Ralph (California)

For an introduction to the Internet, written in plain English rather than computerese, I recommend *An Internet Guide for the Health Professional.*

Advance *magazine, for Respiratory Care Practitioners, February 1997*

I definitely found your book worth reading and will recommend it to my colleagues.

Ulf Sahlin, MD (Sweden)

I will become a passionate propagandist of your books in Southern Africa.

Slava Ryndine, MD (Swaziland, South Africa)

I would not have been able to convince my editor that the Internet is interesting for our readers if I had not read your *Internet Guide*. I owe a lot to you.

French Journalist

An Internet Guide is a helpful book for neophyte browsers or those considering going online...*A Pocket Guide* is an excellent quick reference guide to medical Web sites, newsgroups, and mailing lists.

For the Record *magazine, February 24, 1997*

Exhaustive investigation has gone into *An Internet Guide*; every specialty of importance...is in this volume. Very lucid, and written in an easy-to-understand fashion... *The Pocket Guide* is unique, tiny, convenient enough to fit into a pocket.

The Book Reader, *Fall 1996*

I got the book and it looks fantastic! I've already had several staff members check it out.

Teresa Choi, The Virtual Hospital, University of Iowa

An Internet Guide has been so useful to me this semester. Anyone who has attempted to do any type of web research is painfully aware of how tedious it can be, as well as the tremendous amount of time necessary to find the right site. Your search tips, descriptions of site content, combined with actually having the right URL at my fingertips literally cut hours off my surfing time. I think your book should be on every health care worker's must-buy list.

Dana Rebic, nursing student at Allegheny University (Pennsylvania)

The Internet Workbook for Health Professionals

David Hutchinson, RN

Drawings by Pan

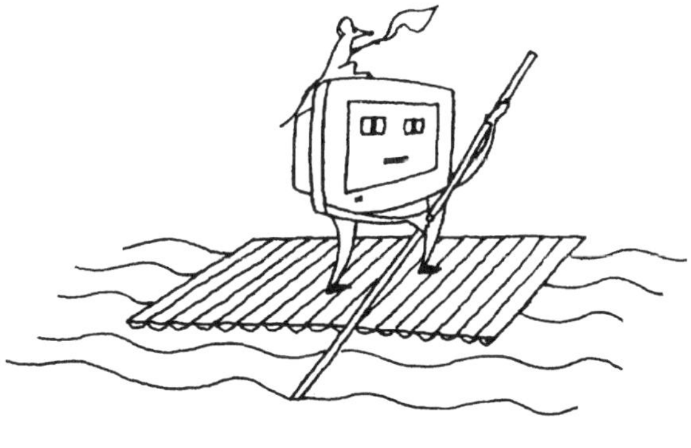

New Wind Publishing

[redacted]

The Internet Workbook for Health Professionals

Graphic Design by Stornetta Publications • storneta@ix.netcom.com

Cataloging Data
Hutchinson, David B.
The Internet Workbook for Health Professionals—1st Ed.
Illustrated, includes bibliography, glossary, and index.
ISBN 0-9651412-4-1

Printed in the United States of America
10 9 8 7 6 5 4 3 2 1

New Wind Publishing

New Wind Publishing
Box 161613
Sacramento, CA 95816-1613
916.451.9039
http://NewWindPub.com
info@NewWindPub.com

Limits of Liability and Disclaimer of Warranty

The author and publisher of this book have used their best efforts in preparing the book. The author and publisher make no warranty of any kind, expressed or implied, with regard to the information contained in this book. The author assumes no responsibility for errors of omissions, nor is any liability assumed for damages resulting from the use of the information contained in this book.

No guarantee is assumed as to the accuracy of information found on any Internet site. The information you find on the Internet should not replace the advice of a trained health professional. If you have any questions about your health, you should always consult a health professional.

Trademarks

Trademarked names appear throughout this book. Rather than list the names and entities that own the trademarks or insert a trademark symbol with each mention of the trademarked names, the publisher states that it is using the names only for editorial purposes and to the benefit of the trademark owner with no intention of infringing upon that trademark.

Acknowledgments

In the greater sense this book was made possible by the thousands of people who have contributed their time and expertise to create the Internet. Many others give their knowledge freely through the Internet via newsgroups, mailing lists, and Web sites. These hardworking people are laying the groundwork for the cultural shift that is to come.

Thanks to those who read through individual sections and corrected my frequent lapses into somnambulism: Jim Hurley, Alok Aurovillian, Terry Vierra, Ping Kwong, Kelly Goudreau, Heather Rebic, Theresa Boschert, Dian Kiser, John Ward, Doug Draper, Susan Zeidenberg, Lynda Lester, Jon Gorrono, Ravi Nemana, and Kathryn Fitzgerald. In particular, Heather, Alok, and Ping made numerous detailed and helpful suggestions.

Jim has tutored me more than anyone in the fine distinctions of the Internet, and has often been willing to explain points at great depth not only to me, but to several online communities as well. He is truly one of the new citizens of the online world.

To Susan I owe a special debt of gratitude for putting up with my beginner's mind and exotic shirts. May she and Bill live a long and happy life together.

Dixie Robertson has been a midwife for all my books, explaining many an obscure point about ink and paper, and her love of publishing has been an inspiration.

Nora Hogan gave me the inestimable gift of goodwill and support when I was still just a newbie to the book world, and for that I will always be in her debt.

Of Pan little needs to be said, since his soul shines forth on every page. Without his artistry this would not be the same book.

Sarah once again came through in quick fashion with a very complex manuscript. I appreciate her cheerfulness and energy in the face of many formatting tangles.

Scotty and Athena made extremely perceptive comments throughout the writing and revising, and even jumped on the keyboard now and again to show that the organic world sports more interesting personalities than any virtual one.

And Marta held the whole together, encouraging the one-pointed writer in me, forcing fluids and rest in the hundred-degree heat of Sacramento summer, and always questioning my semi-colons. Without the enthusiasm and love which we share, this book would not have been possible.

Also by David Hutchinson, RN

- *A Pocket Guide to the Medical Internet* (1997)
- *A Tale of Two Kitties* (1996)
- *An Internet Guide for the Health Professional, Second Edition* (1996) with Michael Hogarth, MD

About the Author

David Hutchinson, RN, BSN, has a degree in physics from Kenyon College, Ohio, and graduated *summa cum laude* from the University of Arizona School of Nursing in 1986. While working as an acute-care nurse in pediatrics at UC Davis Medical Center, Sacramento, CA from 1987 to 1995, he organized orientation materials, wrote a set of quick reference cards for procedures, and developed a unit library.

In 1994 his wife bought a computer to compose music, and David immediately saw the immense potential of the Internet for nurses, and developed a hypertext program for pediatrics and the nursing department. He now teaches computer classes, writes course materials, assists in troubleshooting networks, manages a nursing Web site, and collaborates on numerous projects related to nursing and computers.

In the 90's he began to write for nursing publications, and has contributed several articles on computers, pediatrics, and nursing in general to major nursing journals. To help educate the next generation of nurses and physicians, David lectures to nursing schools and healthcare organizations about the Internet.

Aside from his work in healthcare, David is the devoted father of two well-behaved and well-loved cats, Scotty and Athena, and shares a happy and peaceful home with his feminine half, Marta.

About the Illustrator

Pan Brian Paine was born in England and has pursued a wide-ranging artistic career on both sides of the Atlantic. His works include graphic design, alphabet design, and the restoration of 16th-18th century country houses in England. He also wrote and illustrated four children's books to support the creative development of pre-schoolers. He has held a very successful series of creativity playshops, stimulating a creative spark among the participants.

In recent years his main focus has turned to painting. He has shown mainly in London, San Francisco, Albuquerque, Sedona, and San Diego. His first exhibition was dubbed "The Brushes that Dance with Joy" by a reviewer, which exemplifies Pan's attitude toward his art. He has recently rediscovered a love for illustration, although for years he has been creating innumerable cartoons as a means of relaxation.

Since 1986 Pan has lived at the foot of majestic Mount Shasta in Northern California with his wife Neera, in their unique home, another of his creations.

New Wind Publishing	
Web	http://NewWindPub.com
Email	info@NewWindPub.com
Phone/fax	(916) 451-9039
Postal mail	Box 161613, Sacramento, CA 95816

Contents

Preface

The Internet is like a big swimming pool on a hot summer day, where most of us are standing by the side watching the activities. In one lane are serious athletes, working hard. Next to them are the lap-swimmer wanna-be's who, lacking the stamina to do it alone, swim in relays with the help of friends. In another section of the pool there are kids playing strange games. Still others dive to retrieve treasures from the bottom, and groups toss balls back and forth. Some just lounge by the edge, watching. All have one thing in common: they are having fun in the best place to be on a hot summer day. You would like to join them, but the water looks awfully cold, and you don't know how to swim. "Jump in!" they say. "It's great once you get used to it!" You know they're right, so you take a deep breath...and dip your toe.

In *The Internet Workbook for Health Care Professionals,* author Dave Hutchinson becomes our swimming coach and helps us to participate in all the pool's activities. In Part One: Tools of the Trade, he introduces us to basic computer skills and simple Internet activities such as email. In Part Two: Medical Information, we discover how easy it is to use resources for ourselves or our patients from office, home, or a school computer. In Part Three: Professional Skills, we review ethics and advanced matters regarding our professional use of the Internet.

Eight years of clinical experience as a nurse in pediatrics has made Dave familiar with the needs of patients and staff. He has a strong science background and excellent clinical knowledge, making him able to recognize useful resources on the Web. He loves to teach and adapts his style to the individual, just as he did at the bedside for so many years. He is patient with our anxieties and lets us do it ourselves, and *never* has he said, "I've already explained this to you, don't you remember?"

Dave has lectured in the Nursing Program at California State University in Sacramento for the past year and many students and faculty have also used his books to gain knowledge of how to use the Internet. Although the idea of adding another topic to the curriculum is often met with comments like "I'll learn that next summer when I have time," most students have found that for each hour invested in his books, many hours are saved, as information gathering and dissemination become more efficient.

This Workbook is well designed for the lifestyle of typical health care students and professionals who need knowledge now and don't have a great deal of time to spend obtaining it. Lessons are short and the topics are indexed and organized to allow users to jump to whatever section is of immediate need. A student who needs a literature search for a paper due Monday doesn't have to learn email first. Throughout the book are quick and simple exercises, designed to give hands-on practice and success. Time saving tips, such as reminders to place bookmarks, accompany the practice sessions. It's like having a good friend at your side as you venture out into the unknown waters of the Internet.

Thanks to Dave, our students have become very creative in using the Internet for their nursing education. One, who started the program without ever having used the Net, prepared for a paper about homeless women by conducting an online interview with a shelter resident in another part of the state. A young male student prepared for a debate on breast feeding in public by soliciting opinions from a parents' newsgroup. This semester, for the first time, every student cited a Web reference in their

Teaching-Learning papers. The faculty have set up a mailing list for students in each semester for distribution of grades, announcements and to stimulate discussion outside of class. Each semester we learn something new. Imagine my surprise when I received my first email posting from a student which was linked to a Web page he thought might be interesting for the class to see. I had no idea you could do that!

Never before have I felt more like a beginner next to my students. As their confidence and skills grow, they share new sites and skills with their fellow students and faculty. It has been a bit intimidating to have students who so quickly surpass my own Internet abilities, but as Dave points out in his book, the Internet makes students and teachers out of each of us. At least with his book as a guide, I have a hope of keeping up!

As a writer and teacher, Dave is the finest. He exemplifies how you can be a lifelong student, picking up skills and knowledge in every situation, at every age. He has a wealth of knowledge about the Internet. He is patient. He guides you as a good teacher should, not giving long theoretical lectures, but rather helping you to dive in and get started. Using the Net is a skill you have to do, not just talk about, and Dave understands this.

The first time you pick up the book, you can read any chapter you are interested in, do some short simple exercises, and be successful. On your next lesson Dave will help you go further and achieve additional success. After a few more lessons you will turn around and find that you are swimming by yourself, and it occurs to you that you really don't need your teacher anymore: you have the skills and the confidence to use the Internet by yourself. No greater compliment can ever be paid to a teacher than to have helped students become independent.

So whether you're a toe dipper or a plunger, this book is for you. Come on, let's go for a swim in the info-ocean...

Carolyn VanCouwenberghe, RN, PhD
May, 1997

Clinical Nurse Scientist
UC Davis Medical Center

Professor of Nursing
California State University, Sacramento

Introduction

It is always preferable to have one's face turned toward the future rather than toward the past.

Johann Wolfgang von Goethe

Computers and the Internet are changing so rapidly that it seems impossible for the average person to keep up. Many people buy a computer, get an Internet service provider, and discover that they don't know where to begin. Browsers? Email? Newsgroups? Search engines?

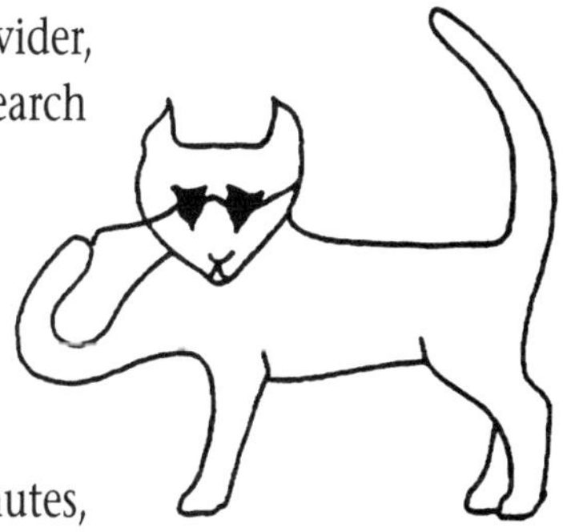

Don't be intimidated. You don't need to be a computer hacker to use the Internet, nor do you need a 500-page listing of sites. Start at the beginning. Sit down at a computer that is connected to the Net, and see what it looks like. Learn a few concepts, then practice. An eight-year-old can learn to navigate the Net in a few minutes, because she takes it as a game, not a set of concepts or some kind of dull "literacy."

This is a hands-on workbook, with an emphasis on medical and health-related resources. It teaches the necessary skills, and in the process takes you on guided journeys into the fascinating world of the medical Internet. Each exercise walks you step-by-step through a basic skill. After completing this book, you will be proficient in email, medical sites on the Web, searching, MEDLINE/CINAHL, and much more. It really can be easy—one step at a time.

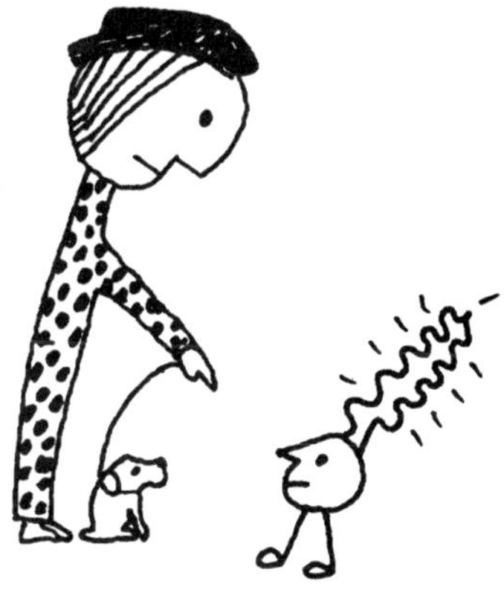

The Internet exemplifies the truth that each person is both student and teacher. You will ask a lot of questions as you learn, and hopefully share your knowledge with others.

In addition to practice, reading about the Internet can be helpful. Rather than publish a gargantuan textbook, in the readings we have used the Internet for source material. This also encourages students to explore and use the Net. Why print it when you can find the same information on the Internet? The Net is overflowing with information about itself.

You don't need any prior experience with the Internet in order to benefit from this workbook, nor do you need any specific hardware or software. However, I do assume that you do have access to the Internet, either at home, in school, or at work.

The text of each chapter introduces the topic. There are three kinds of exercise: Guided Practice, in which basic skills are shown step-by-step; Problem-Solving, in which these skills can be tried without explicit directions; and Thought and Discussion, in which issues and ideas are explored. At the end of each chapter are online readings.

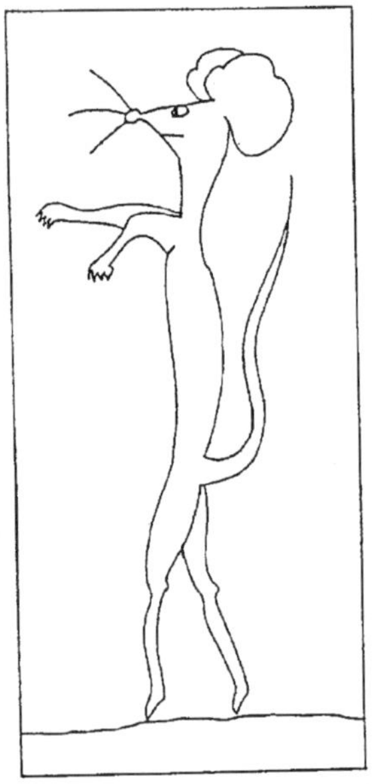

The exercises and readings in this book are not specific to Windows, Macintosh, or Unix computers and programs. Using the Internet does not require a specific program or operating system. But in order to give specific exercises, I have chosen those programs which the majority of people are actually using: Netscape Navigator, Eudora, and Internet Explorer. Where Netscape Navigator and Internet Explorer differ, the Guided Exercises explain the procedure for both. Throughout the book I follow the common usage of "Netscape" to refer to the browser program (Navigator) which the Netscape Corporation produces.

The Internet can seem overwhelmingly complex, but in fact you will learn it the same way you learn anything else, step by step. The basic skills are not difficult, and working through the book chapter by chapter gives a practical and thorough grasp of them. Without even trying, you will morph into a nurse nerd, and wonder what the fuss was all about.

This workbook is based on hundreds of hours teaching classes, giving one-to-one tutorials, and demonstrating computers and the Internet. In addition I have written dozens of teaching handouts, several articles, and two books (*An Internet Guide for the Health Professional* and *A Pocket Guide to the Medical Internet*) in the last year, in an attempt to give the best resources to health professionals. If you are interested in these books, see the back page for an order form.

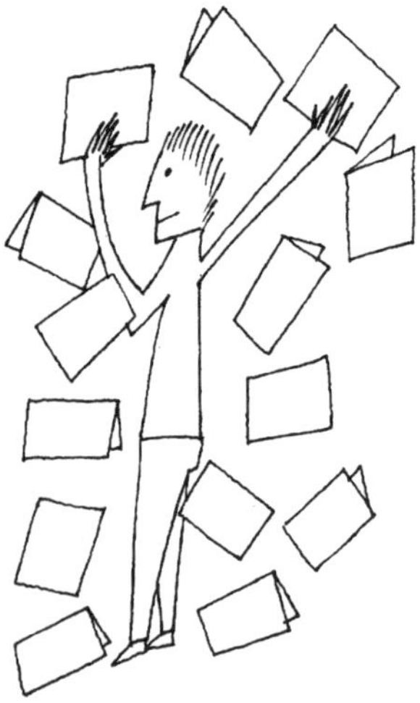

Training in any of the health professions involves years of education, during which time you master an immense vocabulary and set of concepts. You already are an "information specialist." But medical knowledge is progressive, and despite the competence you have on graduation, you have to keep up with changes.

Healthcare workers have a general disdain for computers, a feeling I shared only a few years ago. But the Internet is different than the clunky mainframe systems most of us grew up with: exciting things are happening! I wrote this book because this phenomenal medical resource goes unused by too many physicians and nurses. It is a global library, newsstand, meeting room, and university, drawing patients and healthcare workers closer together as we educate and learn from one another. Once we learn to use it, we can communicate with professionals around the world, keep informed of the rapid changes in medical knowledge and practice, and improve the public health.

We live in dynamic times. Bertrand Russell says: "The gulf separating man from his past has widened from generation to generation, and finally from decade to decade." A new world is forming, one that is going to transform health care in a very few years, and we can all help to guide and create the healthcare info-space of the 21st century.

Typographic Conventions in this Book

Text:

- Acronyms are upper-case: FTP, HTML, CINAHL

Guided Exercises:

- Each letter (A, B, C) signifies an independent exercise
- Text you should type is in `Courier Font`
- Anything you should click is underlined, including <u>menu items</u>, <u>buttons,</u> <u>hypertext links</u>, or <u>icons</u>
- Menu items are separated by commas: "Click <u>File</u>, <u>Print</u>" means to click the File menu item, then Print

Tables:

- If a URL covers two lines, the first line ends with a slash (/)

Glossary:

- Letters of words that form acronyms are underlined:
  <u>F</u>ile <u>T</u>ransfer <u>P</u>rotocol

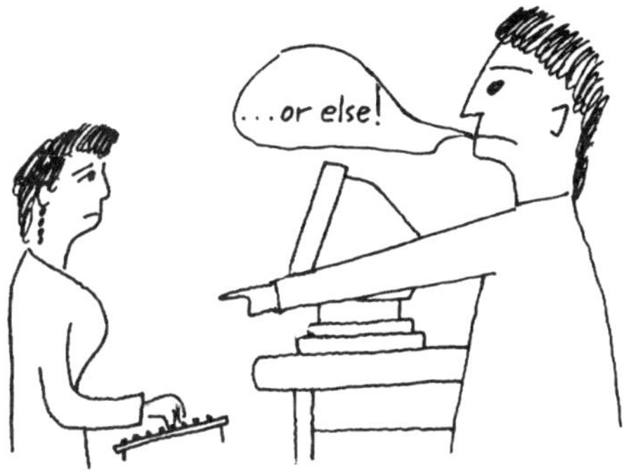

What You Will Not Find in This Book

Whereof one cannot speak, theron one must remain silent.
Ludwig Wittgenstein, Tractatus Logico-Philosophicus

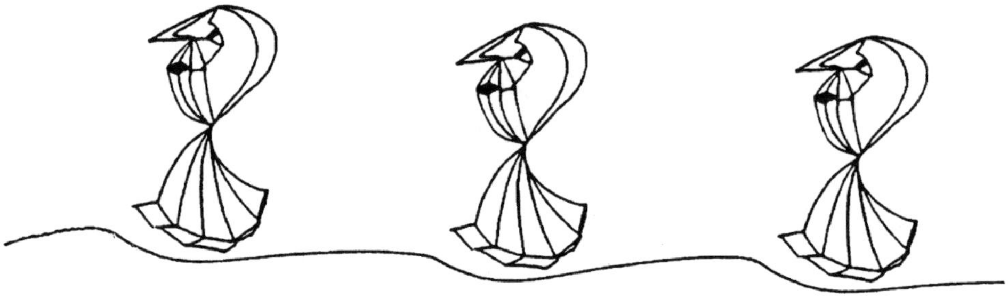

There are many aspects of computers and the Internet that you should <u>not</u> spend time on in the beginning, because they will only distract from learning the basics. The following lists topics to ignore for now (e.g. creating graphics) or delegate to a paid professional (e.g. setting up Windows 95 for networking.)

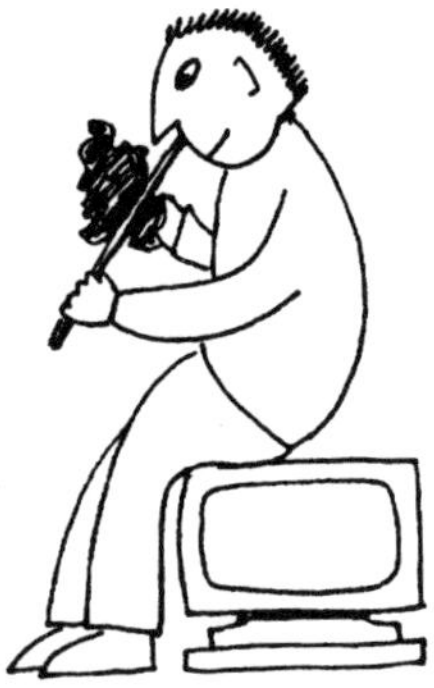

Fiddling with your OS

Topics NOT covered in this book:

- How to set up Windows 95 or Windows 3.1 for the Internet
- How to use different operating systems
- How to upgrade or fix a computer
- How to write programs
- How to create a Web page or site
- How to create graphics, multimedia, or video
- How to play games on a computer or the Internet
- How to use mainframe hospital computer systems
- How to use clinical information systems or electronic medical records

Part One:
Tools of the Trade

No Experience Necessary
Windows and Your Computer
Browsers and the Web
Anatomy of a Web Site
Electronic Mail
Bookmarks: Beam Me Back, Scotty!

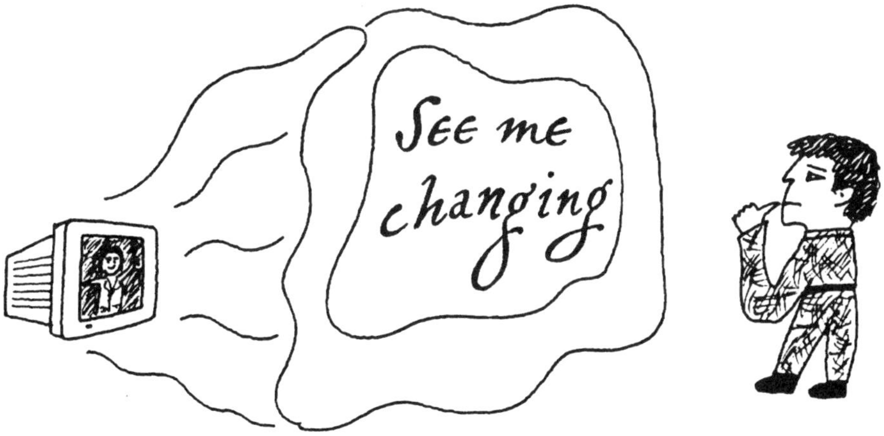

After finishing Part One, you will be able to:

- *Browse the Internet*
- *Start a program*
- *Save a file*
- *Move between two programs*
- *Use Netscape Navigator or Microsoft Explorer*
- *Send and receive electronic mail*
- *Use Eudora email*
- *Save Internet sites to a bookmark list and organize them*

Chapter 1: No Experience Necessary

I never lose an opportunity of urging a practical beginning, however small, for it is wonderful how often the mustard seed germinates and roots itself.

Florence Nightingale

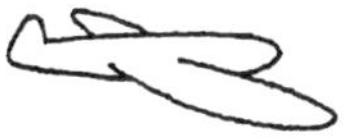

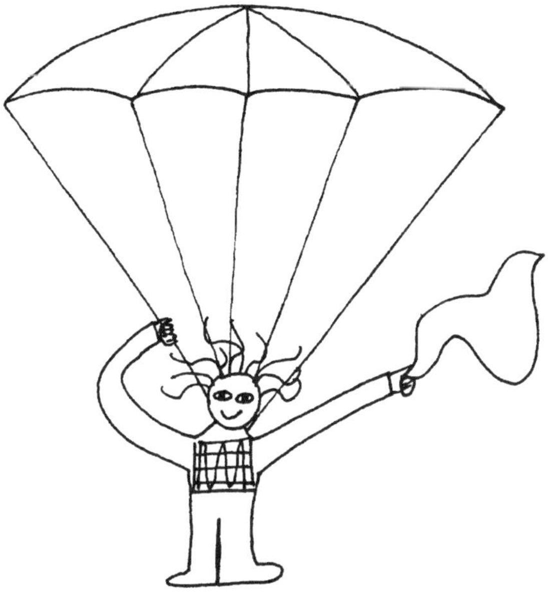

IN THIS CHAPTER

browser
double-click
home page
hypertext
Internet
link
menu bar
mouse
scrolling
URL
World Wide Web

For most people the biggest obstacle to using the Internet is an irrational anxiety about the unknown, and the best solution is to have a friend take five minutes to teach the basics. Do that, and the looming Internet phantom will vanish.

Internet

A worldwide collection of computers that communicate with each other.

Books are mainly useful as references. Experiment, play around, explore, ask a few questions, and you will soon move beyond them.

Your classroom should have computers with access to the Internet, and a browser program such as Netscape should be up and running. For this first lesson it's not necessary to know how to start a program, flip floppies, or boggle the bots. That comes later.

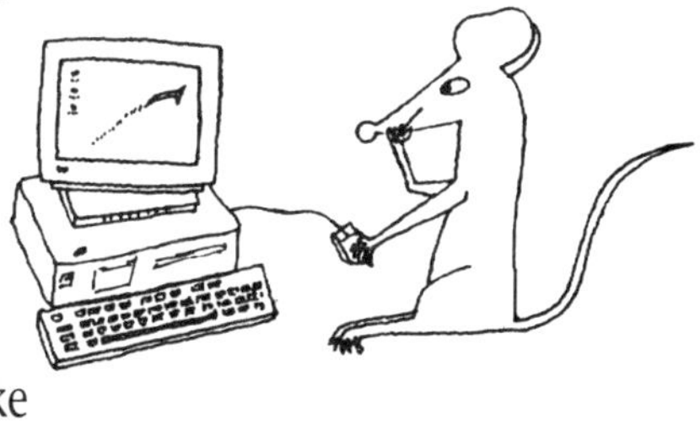

Next to the computer is a mouse. When you move it across the pad, you will see an arrow on the screen move at the same time. The mouse pointer is used to make choices on a computer.

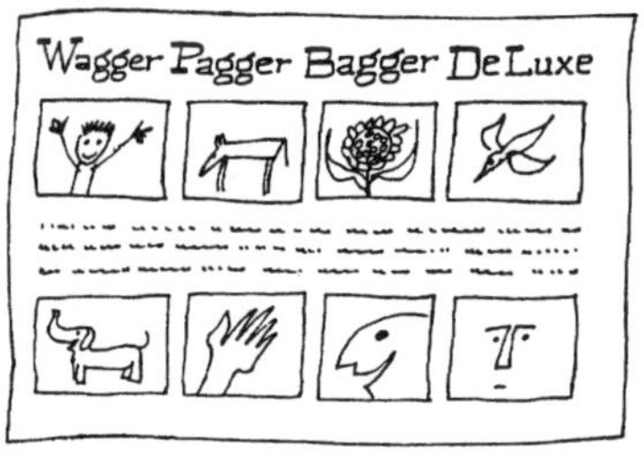

On the screen is a Web page, probably the home page for your school or organization. A Web page is just a computerized document with words and pictures. Some of the words on the screen should be underlined, meaning that they are links to other documents. Move the mouse so that the arrow is over one of the underlined words; the arrow should turn into an image of a pointing hand. Now, while the pointer is still on top of the word, and looking at the screen, click once with your index finger on the left-side button of the mouse.

The onscreen pointer will change to an image of an hourglass for a second or three, and then another Web page will appear. The page may appear very fast, or it may arrive in pieces, one picture filling in first, then another, and another.

Single click, double click?

Double-clicking means to click the mouse twice, quickly.

Welcome to the Net! Breathe deep: you have just surfed the World Wide Web, using a hypertext link. You've joined the millions of people exploring the new info-world. In a short time you will be able to find books, discussions, news, entertainment, shopping—just about anything.

Hypertext

A hypertext document has computer-activated links to other documents.

Try clicking on any underlined word on the screen. Take five minutes and practice moving from page to page. Don't worry about getting lost, destroying the computer, or accidentally infiltrating the CIA. That comes later.

Navigation

How do you get back to the first screen? Toward the top of the screen will be a picture of a house, with the word Home underneath it. Click once on the house, and the starting (Home) page should reappear.

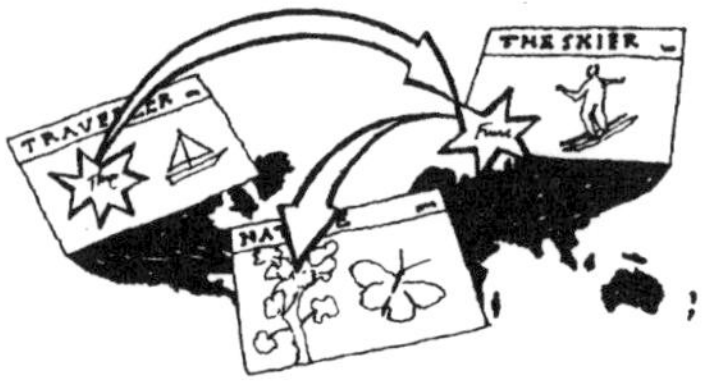

After visiting a few pages, go back to them by using the onscreen button to the left of the house which has the word Back underneath it. Clicking on this several times will retrace the journey in reverse, and end at the Home page.

Above the Home and Back buttons you see a list of words: File, Edit, Go...Help. This line of words is called the menu bar. Move the onscreen arrow over the word Go and click once. A list of the documents you have already visited will drop down. Click the name of any document to return to it.

Menu

A list of choices that appears when you click an onscreen word.

Scrolling

Often the contents of a Web page continue below the bottom of the screen, so that the document is more like a continuous scroll than a piece of paper. The easiest way to see what is below is to use the keyboard button which says PgDn (PageDown). When you tap this key once, the program moves down one screen. Be sure to tap the key quickly rather than hold it down; if you hold it, the program will very quickly scroll through several pages of information, and unless you have Data's positronic brain, you will miss everything. To move up, tap the PgUp (Page Up) key.

Web Addresses

Below the onscreen button bar is an area that shows the location of the current Web page. Every document on the Internet has an address, just as every house in the world has its own address. Look at a fictional address:

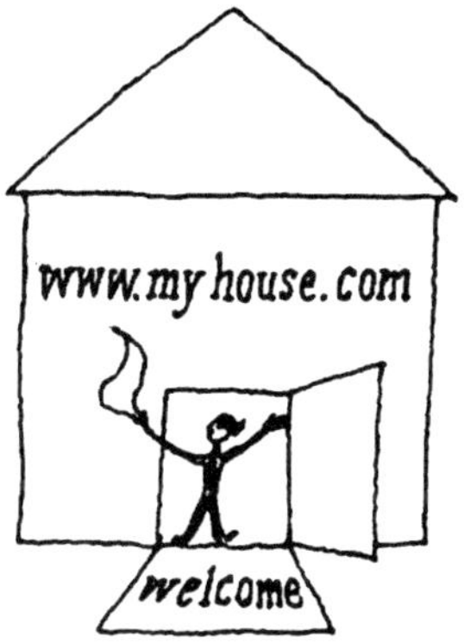

John P.
Apartment 2
22 First St.
Anytown, USA

The information reads from smallest to largest, starting with the apartment and ending with the country. What if we were to write the address on one line, instead of several lines, putting a slash between each linc?

JohnP/Apartment2/22FirstStreet/Anytown/USA

How would it look if we reversed the order?

USA/Anytown/22FirstStreet/Apartment2/JohnP

This way of writing an address reads from largest to smallest, but the information is still understandable.

An Internet address, called a URL (Uniform Resource Locator), is written like this last example, except that instead of pointing to a physical house, it points to a site on the Internet. Here is the Internet address for the CDC journal *Emerging Infectious Diseases*:

http://www.cdc.gov/ncidod/EID/eid.htm

How to Speak Keyboard

@	at
.	dot
/	slash
~	tilde
_	underscore

You can go to a document by typing the URL into the location area of your browser, just as you would call a person on the telephone by dialing a phone number. ***You don't have to type the "http://" which is in front of the address.***

Here's another time-saver. Try clicking once in the location bar, type `rxlist`, and press the Enter key. Surprise! If the address has www in front and com at the end, Netscape will fill in the remainder. The complete address for this document is: http://www.rxlist.com, a pharmacology site with medication dosage, effects, interactions, and contraindications.

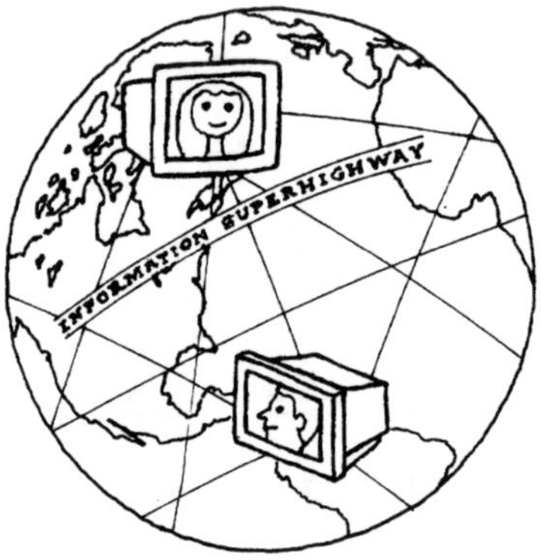

A Quick History of the Net

The Internet is the sum of all the computers, information, and people which today forms a worldwide network. You will hear it referred to as Cyberspace, the Net, or the Information Superhighway, all of which refer to the same thing. It began in the 1960's, its technology was developed in the 70's, universities used it in the 80's, and business has dominated it in the 90's. What will happen to it in the next decade is anybody's guess.

Network
Two or more computers which can send information back and forth.

Using the Internet, you can find and print documents, send electronic mail, and publish your own information electronically. You can watch a video, place a telephone call, send a fax, buy things, and play interactive games. There are perhaps one hundred million people using the Net at the current time. The size of the Internet in several dimensions (the number of computers connected, the number of documents available, the number of people using it) has been doubling every six to twelve months since it began. In other words, it is growing exponentially, with no end in sight, which makes its future very unpredictable. This is why people are so excited, and so apprehensive.

No single corporation or country owns the Internet or dictates how it can be used. A variety of committees of the Internet Society (http://www.isoc.org), a voluntary organization, develops international standards for the way information is exchanged. The Internet has developed over time by consensus, testing, and the free exchange of knowledge.

In addition to the many medical sites you will visit as you work through this book, you will find an infinite variety of non-medical sites. Even for the dedicated workaholic, a few minutes' dawdling is permitted.

Only the Beginning...

Amazon.com	http://www.amazon.com	Over one million books to buy online.
Biography.com	http://www.biography.com	In case you've forgotten Montaigne or Montana.
Cable News Network	http://www.cnn.com	Background, links, related stories.
City.net	http://www.city.net	Over five thousand worldwide destinations.
Discovery Channel	http://www.discovery.com	The infinite world, explained anew.
Epicurious	http://www.epicurious.com	Click and cook.
HyperHistory	http://www.hyperhistory.com	The world that was. Go to HyperHistory Online.
iMusic	http://www.imusic.com	Rock and roll is here to stay.
Map Quest	http://www.mapquest.com	The whole world's waiting.
Maps On Us	http://www.mapsonus.com	Plan your trip. Maps, directions.
Movie Database	http://us.imdb.com	Everything about celluloid dreams.
MSNBC	http://www.msnbc.com	Joint production by NBC and Microsoft.
Pathfinder	http://www.pathfinder.com	Time-Warner's gigantic media site.
Project Gutenberg	http://www.promo.net/pg	One thousand books online; more to come.
Reference Desk	http://thorplus.lib.purdue.edu/ reference	Government, dictionaries, maps, science.
Rent.net	http://www.rent.net	More than one million apartments.
Virtual Tours	http://www.dreamscape.com/ frankvad/tours.html	Visit 200 museums, 100 cities, and more.
Weather Channel	http://www.weather.com	Find out if it's raining before you get there.
Why Files	http://whyfiles.news.wisc.edu	Everybody's favorite question: Why?
World Wide Arts	http://wwar.com	All the arts: film, books, museums, dance.
Women's Resources	http://sunsite.unc.edu/cheryb/ women/wresources.html	Links and more links. Wonderful place to find out what's happened in the last 30 years.

EXERCISES

Each lettered exercise is independent.
(Links available at http://NewWindPub.com/workbook)

A note on Netscape Navigator and Microsoft Internet Explorer:

Exercises in this book are written primarily for Netscape Navigator, versions 3 and 4, because it is the most widely used browser. Differences between these versions, or between Navigator and Explorer, are noted in parentheses.

I. Guided Practice

A. FORWARD, BACK, HOME BUTTONS

1. Start Netscape or Explorer.
2. Click any underlined word. This will take you to a new page.
3. Click any underlined word on this page. This will take you to a third page.
4. Along the top of the program window are a series of buttons: Back, Forward, Home, etc. Click the Home button to return to your starting (Home) page.
5. Click the Back button. You will return to the page you just saw.
6. Click the Back button again. In this way you can retrace a path through a series of Web pages.

B. GO MENU

1. Along the top of the Netscape window you see the series of words: File, Edit, View, Go. Click once on the word Go.
2. You should see a list of pages you have visited. Click any page to go there.

C. TYPE AN ADDRESS: LOCATION BAR

1. Beneath the button bar you should see a narrow text area with a Web address of the page you are looking at (http://...) (If this bar is not showing, click Options, Show Location (Netscape 4: View, Show Location Toolbar; Explorer: Click the word Address beneath the Back button.)
2. Click once inside the Location bar. The entire address should reverse colors, with white letters on a navy blue background.
3. Type `www.cdc.gov` and press the Enter key to visit the Centers for Disease Control. You must type the letters exactly, and have the periods (dots) there also.
4. Note that you don't have to type the prefix http://

D. TYPE AN ADDRESS: FILE MENU

You can also use the File menu to get to a page by typing its address.

1. Click the word File along the top of the Netscape window. A menu of choices drops down.
2. Click Open Location (Netscape 4: Open Page; Explorer: Open)
3. Type `cnn` and press the Enter key.
4. Note that the address you go to is www.cnn.com For commercial sites that start with "www" and end with "com" you can simply type the part in the middle, and Netscape will supply the rest. (Explorer does not have this function.)

E. VISIT NETSCAPE'S HOME PAGE

1. Click once on the large letter N in the upper right of the Netscape window. This will take you to Netscape's home page. If you are running Explorer, go to http://home.netscape.com
2. Click the words Guide to Internet on the lower left of the picture at the top of the page.
3. Press the Page Down (or PgDn) and Page Up (or PgUp) keys to move down and up the page.
4. On the navigation bar near the top of the page (Guide, Business, Computers, Entertainment...), click the Entertainment tab.

F. SEARCH FOR A WORD ON A WEB PAGE

1. Go to the Entertainment page from the last exercise, if you are not already there.
2. Click the word Edit in the Netscape menu (File, Edit, View, etc.) and then click Find.
3. Type humor and press the Enter key.

4. Close the Find window by clicking on the Cancel button. The word search should have found the Humor section lower down on the Entertainment page.

G. RIGHT-CLICK

1. Right-click any Web page.
2. Click the Back selection to go back, or on Forward to go forward.
3. (This function is not available in Explorer.)

H. ADD A BOOKMARK

(See Chapter 6 for more exercises with bookmarks.)

1. Click the Home button to return to your home page.
2. Click any underlined link.
3. Click the menu Bookmarks, Add Bookmark (Explorer: Favorites, Add to Favorites)
4. Click the Home button to return to your home page.
5. Click Bookmarks (Explorer: Favorites) then click the item you added. Note that the browser takes you to that page.

II. Problem-Solving

- Explore Netscape's help manual. Click the Help menu item at the far right of the menu bar and see if you can use it to learn about the Netscape program or the Internet.
- Go to Yahoo (http://www.yahoo.com), find the Health section, and read the summary paragraphs about today's health news.
- Go to Amazon.com (http://www.amazon.com) and try to find a book on the medical Internet.

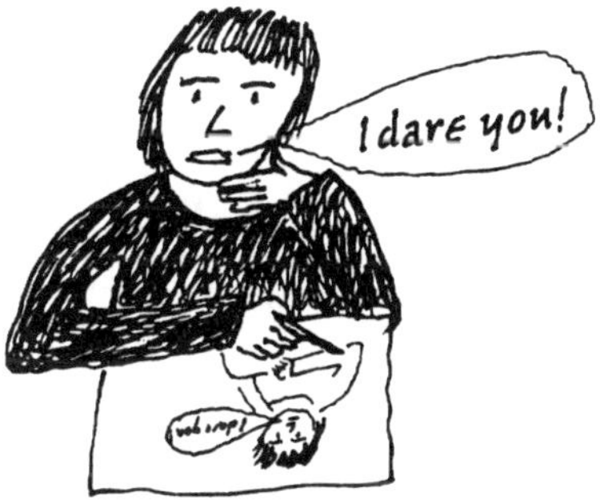

III. Thought and Discussion

- What effect do the drawings in this book have on your understanding of the information presented here?
- Describe to another person "where" you were on the Web.
- What is the difference between a television program and a Web page in terms of who is presenting the information and what you do while you are seeing it?

Readings From the Net

(Links available at http://NewWindPub.com/workbook)

Introductions to the Internet

Beginners Central	http://www.northernwebs.com/bc/begin00.html	Simple language. Good introduction to the Internet.
The December List	http://www.december.com	Go to Internet Web or CMC info sources.
Guide to Cyberspace	http://www.eit.com/web/www.guide	Dated, but still an excellent description.
Internet 101	http://www.impactonline.org/internet	Short, well-organized, practical.
Internet Starter Kit	http://www.mcp.com/23663274807484/hayden/iskm/book.html	Entire text of the third edition. Macintosh and Windows versions.
Internet Timeline	http://info.isoc.org/guest/zakon/Internet/History/HIT.html	A quick historical view, from the formation of ARPA in 1957 to the present.
Internet History	http://info.isoc.org/internet-history	A longer hypertext version of the above.
Learn The Net	http://learnthenet.com	Friendly, short introductions.
Origins of the World Wide Web	http://homepage.seas.upenn.edu/~lzeltser/WWW	By Lenny Zeltser. Short introduction to the origins of the Web, browsers, and hypertext.
World Wide Web	http://www.w3.org/pub/WWW/WWW	From the World Wide Web consortium.

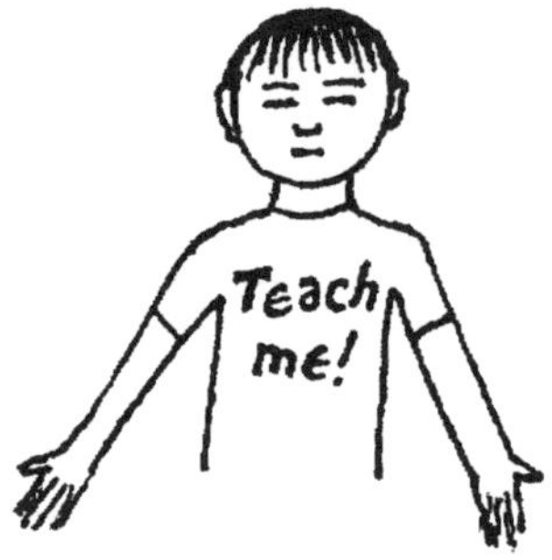

Chapter 2: Windows and Your Computer

He had been eight years upon a project for extracting sunbeams out of cucumbers...

Jonathan Swift, Voyage to Laputa

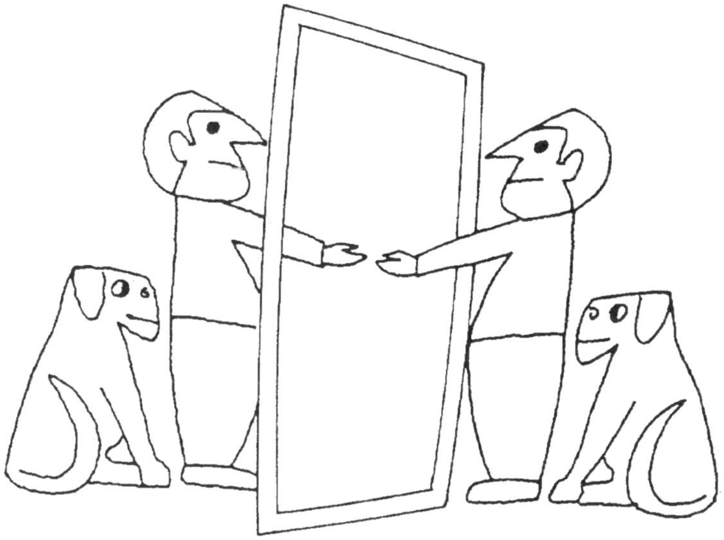

IN THIS CHAPTER

cursor
desktop
disk
double-click
file
floppy
GUI
hard disk
icon
memory
microcomputer
operating system
PC
program
shortcut
software
window

Operating System

Windows, produced by the Microsoft Corporation, is the name for the most common operating system in use with personal computers. An operating system controls all the physical components of a computer (keyboard, mouse, printer), the way programs interact and look, and the way information is moved between physical devices or stored on disk. The operating system is a hardworking fellow, not at all the ogre we saw in the movie Tron.

Periodically an upgraded version of an operating system or program becomes available. You can continue to use the old version or buy the new one. The new version will be different in some aspects, but often works very much like the previous one. New programs often require newer computers in order to run well. Now you see why the lifetime of the average computer is three years.

Most personal computers today use the Microsoft Windows operating system, either Windows 3.1 or Windows 95. If you are familiar with either one of these, you should have no trouble with the other. (The first version of this operating system was called DOS; this year's version is called Windows 97.)

Desktop

The desktop is the computer screen which shows (after the arcane DOS messages) when you turn on your computer. Your physical desk holds items such as a calendar, an article you are writing, paper, or a dictionary. By analogy, on the desktop of a computer you can organize programs or documents you are working with.

> **Icon**
>
> A small picture used to signify a program, file, or function.

Windows 3.1

When you start Windows 3.1 it displays the Program Manager, which shows pictures, called icons, for the different programs in your computer. The icons are arranged into groups, such as Applications or Accessories.

Windows 95

When you start Windows 95, you will see a bar across the bottom of the screen with the word Start on the lower left. You may also see pictures for various programs or documents, such as My Computer or Explorer.

Starting and Closing a Program

In both Windows 3.1 and Windows 95 you start a program by double-clicking on the icon for that program. Depending on how fast your computer is, it may take a few seconds or as much as a minute or two for a program to start. Go ahead and start the Netscape program.

There are several different ways to close a program. Along the top of most programs is a line of words called the menu bar. When you Click the word File you will see the word Exit at the bottom of the list. Clicking on Exit will close the program. You can also Click the upper left of the window that a program is in, and a menu will appear with the word Close at the bottom. Clicking on this will also close the program. Try closing and restarting Netscape.

Programs and Files

Software is another word for program. (Programs are also referred to as applications, accessories, utilities, gewgaws, gimcracks, and *cool stuff.*) You use a program to accomplish a specific task, such as to send email, browse the World Wide Web, type documents, or create a teaching presentation. Each program is designed to do one thing, but the trend over the last few years has been for each program to include more and more functions. You can use the Netscape browser, for example, to send and receive email, create a Web page, read discussion groups, download files, keep a calendar, and create a project list. A few years ago each of these tasks required a separate program.

A file is a document in the computer. Each program will have many files that come with it, so your computer's hard drive will have a lot of files even when it is new. (In fact, it is common for much of the hard drive space to be taken up with the operating system and programs.)

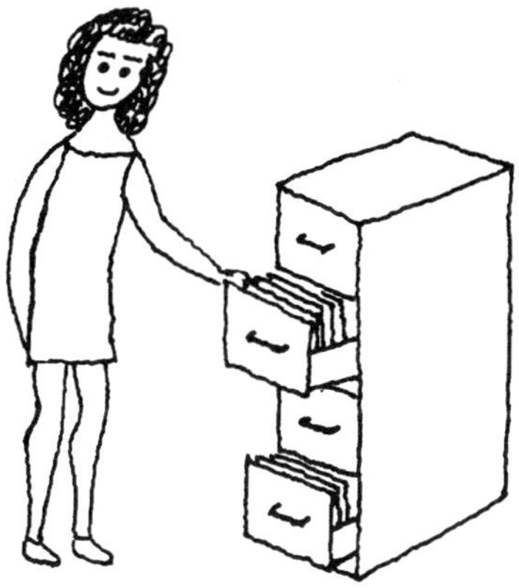

After you create a document (see Chapter 17) you then save it as a file onto the hard drive of the computer. Hard drives today have an enormous amount of space, as measured in terms of text: a two gigabyte (GB) hard drive can hold the equivalent of two thousand novels.

File Manager and Explorer

File
A document saved in a computer.

After a while you will have created a number of files with your computer. The File Manager (Windows 3.1) or the Explorer (Windows 95) are built-in programs for finding, organizing, sorting, naming, moving, and deleting files. If you think of your hard drive as a filing cabinet, the files are organized into separate folders, called directories. A computer directory can have sub-directories, and sub-sub-directories. (If musicians created computers, would they be hemi-demi-semi-directories?)

Hard Disk and Memory

When you start a program, you hear the hard drive rotating inside the case. The hard drive is a series of magnetic disks which store the information inside your computer. When a program starts, an electronic copy of the program is copied from the hard drive to a temporary holding area called RAM (random access memory). RAM uses electronic chips rather than a spinning disk, so it can work with information about a thousand times faster than the hard drive. By putting the program in RAM while it is running, the computer can thus operate much faster. This is the reason that a computer needs to have an adequate amount of RAM for the programs it will run.

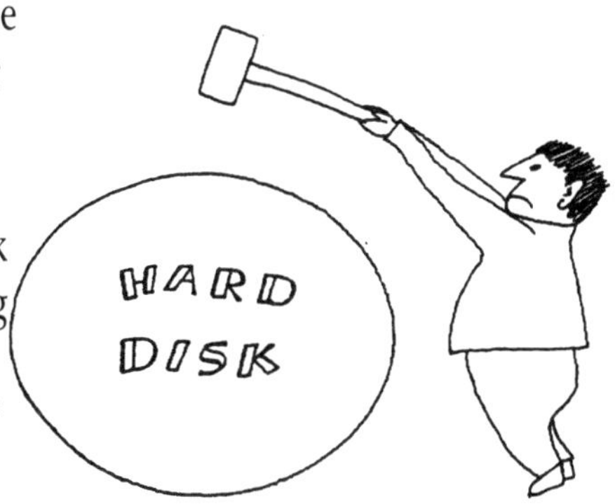

Central Processing Unit (CPU)

Although a computer has many chips, the CPU is the main chip which works with information. In general a computer is named after the CPU: we refer to it as a "486" or a "Pentium." Each type of chip has different models which run at different speeds, measured in megahertz (millions of cycles per second). When you see a computer referred to as a Pentium 133, it means that it can process 133 million instructions per second.

The two physical parts of your computer that determine how fast it will work are RAM and the CPU. With more RAM and a faster CPU, programs will start faster, operate more smoothly, and have fewer problems.

Modem

A device which converts information to a form that can travel over telephone lines.

Other Components

A typical computer has a monitor, keyboard, mouse, case, and printer. Inside the case are the modem, hard drive, floppy drive, power supply, and other components.

For a computer to connect to the Internet it must have a means to send and receive information, either a modem (if it is sending information over a telephone line) or a network card (if it is attached to a network). Other devices can be added, such as a card for viewing television, for hearing radio, or for playing stereo-quality sound.

A printer is attached to most computers, so you can print a paper copy of documents. Advanced printers can also make copies and scan paper documents into electronic form.

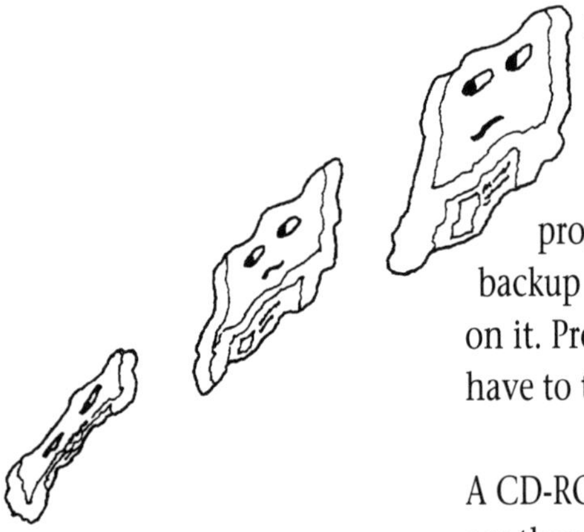

A floppy disk, like the hard disk, stores information in magnetic form. You insert a floppy disk into the slot in the front of the case, then use a program to save or move a file to the floppy. In this way you can make a backup copy of the information, or take the file to a separate computer to work on it. Programs themselves are sold on floppy disks; before you can use them you have to transfer the program from the disks to the hard drive. This is fairly easy.

A CD-ROM (CD, compact disk) stores information as bumps on the disk, which are then read by a laser beam. CD's hold much more information than a floppy—about 600 megabytes, compared to 1.4 megabytes for a floppy. For this reason, large programs usually come on CD-ROM. Games, reference texts, or encyclopedias, which require a large amount of information, come on CD-ROM. A newer version of CD-ROM disks, called DVD (digital video disks) will be able to hold much more information, 4.7 to 17 gigabytes (4,700 to 17,000 megabytes) on a disk the same size. This will enable an entire movie to be placed on a CD.

If computers continue to advance so rapidly, in a very few years they will be able to translate speech, analyze handwriting, edit movies, and much more.

EXERCISES

Each lettered exercise is independent.
(Links available at http://NewWindPub.com/workbook)

I. Guided Practice

Windows 3.1

A. OPEN A PROGRAM GROUP AND START A PROGRAM

1. In the program manager, Click the Window menu item.
2. Click Accessories.
3. In the Accessories window, double-click Write. (If double-clicking is difficult, click once and press the Enter key.) This is the MS Write word processor.

ENLARGE A PROGRAM TO FULL SCREEN

1. If the Write program does not occupy the entire screen, double-click the title bar (the strip across the top where you see MS Write.)
2. To return the window to its previous size, double-click the bar again.

SAVE A DOCUMENT

1. Type a few letters.
2. Click File, then Save.
3. Type the word `junk` (With Windows 3.1, file names are limited to 8 letters. You cannot use spaces.)
4. Click OK. The program will add the three-letter extension .wri to the end, so the whole file name is now junk.wri

CLOSE A PROGRAM

1. Click the square in the upper left of the Write window.
2. Click Close.

OPEN A DOCUMENT

1. Close Write. Click File, Exit.
2. Open MS Write again.
3. Click File, Open.
4. Click once on the file named junk.wri
5. Click OK.

PRINT A DOCUMENT

1. Click File, Print.
2. Click OK in the box which pops up.

B. SWITCH BETWEEN PROGRAMS

You can use the two keys Alt and Tab to quickly move between two programs that are running on your computer at the same time.

1. Click the small triangle pointing down in the upper right of the Write window. The window will either disappear or shrink down to a small icon at the bottom of the screen.
2. Double-click the program titled Paintbrush in the Accessories group.
3. Hold down the Alt key with your left thumb.
4. Tap the Tab key, keeping the Alt key depressed. Do not hold down the Tab key, but simply tap it quickly.
5. In the middle of the screen a small window will appear.
6. If you do not see Write in the window, tap the Tab key again. Keep the Alt key depressed.
7. When you see the Write program, let go of the Alt key. The Write program will pop up on the screen.
8. Now hold down Alt and tap Tab to return to the Paintbrush program.

C. MOVE FILES

In this exercise you copy a file to a floppy disk.

1. Put a floppy disk in the slot in the front of the computer. It will only fit one way; if it doesn't go in, turn the floppy over and try again. Be sure to insert the end with the metal tab.
2. Click the Window menu.
3. Click Main.
4. Double-click (or click and press the Enter key) on File Manager. The picture looks like a filing cabinet.
5. Along the top you see letters a, b, c, etc. Click once on c to make sure you are looking at the hard drive of your computer.
6. On the left are directories (areas in the computer). On the right are files.
7. Use the arrow key or Page Down key to move down the list of directories. As each directory is highlighted, the files in that area show up on the right side of the screen.
8. Go to the Windows directory and click once on its name in the left side of the screen.

9. Click the View menu, then on Sort by Name.
10. Along the bottom of the right hand side of the screen is a scroll bar. Click the darker part of this area and hold down your finger. Drag this bar to the right until you see the file junk.wri
11. Click once on the name of the file. Be careful not to click twice, or the program will start.
12. Click File, then Copy.
13. Type `a:` (the letter a with a colon after it) and click OK (or press the Enter key). The light by the floppy disk slot will come on, showing that the file is being copied.

DRAG AND DROP A FILE

1. Another way to copy a file is by dragging it. Click the file junk.wri and keep your finger held down.
2. Drag the file across the screen. The pointer will look like an arrow with a small piece of paper behind it.
3. When the pointer is over the letter a in the upper left of the screen, let go of the mouse button.
4. If a window pops up "Are you sure you want to copy the files..." Click Yes.
5. A window will pop up "Confirm file replace..." The computer recognizes that the file junk.wri is already on the floppy. Click No to cancel this operation.

RENAME A FILE

1. Click the drive letter a in the upper left of the File Manager window.
2. Click once on the file junk.wri in the right side of the screen.
3. Click the menu File, then Rename.
4. Type `junk2.wri` and click OK.

COPY A FILE FROM A FLOPPY TO THE HARD DRIVE

1. Double-click the drive letter c in the upper left of the File Manager window.
2. Click the Window menu, then Tile Horizontally. You should now see both a and c drives on the screen.
3. If you cannot see the Windows folder in the c drive window, scroll until it is visible.
4. Click the file junk2.wri and, keeping your finger held down, drag the file over to the Windows folder. Drop it on the folder.
5. Double-click the title bar of the c drive window (where you see c:\...) to expand this window.
6. Click the Window menu, then Refresh so the file list will be updated.
7. Scroll over and look for junk2.wri

FIND A FILE

1. Scroll up and click c:\ on the left side of the window.
2. Click File, then Search.
3. Type `junk2.wri` and press the Enter key. Wait a minute as the computer looks for the file.

DELETE A FILE

1. Click the drive letter a.
2. Click the name of the file junk2.wri
3. Click the File menu, then Delete. (Or press the Delete key.)
4. Click OK.

Windows 95

Windows 95 has many ways to do most simple functions. We will only cover a few.

D. START A PROGRAM

Open a program group and start a program

1. Click the Start button in the lower left of the screen.
2. Move the mouse until it points to Programs.
3. In the list that pops up, move the mouse until it points to Accessories.
4. In the list that pops up, move the mouse until it points to WordPad and Click it. WordPad is the successor to Write.

ENLARGE A PROGRAM TO FULL SCREEN

1. Same as Windows 3.1

SAVE A DOCUMENT

1. Same as Windows 3.1, except file names can have up to 256 letters, and spaces are allowed. The file will get the three-letter extension .doc with WordPad.

CLOSE A PROGRAM

1. Same as Windows 3.1, except the square in the upper left has been replaced by an icon of the program.

OPEN A DOCUMENT

1. Same as Windows 3.1

PRINT A DOCUMENT

1. Same as Windows 3.1

E. SWITCH BETWEEN PROGRAMS

1. Same as Windows 3.1, except when you use Alt + Tab you will see small icons of all the programs, rather than one at a time. You will see a box around the icon of the program that will pop up when you release the Tab key.

F. MOVE FILES

In this exercise you copy a file to a floppy disk.

1. Put a floppy disk in the slot in the front of the case. It will only fit one way; if it doesn't go in, turn the floppy over and try again. Be sure to insert the end with the metal tab.
2. Right-click the Start button.
3. Click Explore. This starts the Windows Explorer, the successor to the File Manager. The functions are the same, but the windows looks different.
4. Click the gray scroll bar in the middle of the screen and drag it to the top.
5. Click the plus (+) or minus (-) signs in the left side of the screen to expand or contract the listing of directories in an area. Try this with the drive letter C: a few times until you understand visually what is happening.
6. Use the arrow key or Page Down key to move down the list of directories. As each directory is highlighted, the files in that area show up on the right side of the screen.
7. Go to the Windows directory and click once on its name in the left side of the screen.
8. Click the View menu, then Arrange Icons, then by Name.
9. Click the View menu, then List.
10. Along the bottom of the right hand side of the screen is a scroll bar. Click the darker part of this area and hold down your finger. Drag this bar to the right until you see the file junk.wri
11. Right-click the name of the file.
12. Move the mouse over Send To, then click 3½ Floppy (A)

DRAG AND DROP A FILE

1. Same as Windows 3.1

RENAME A FILE

1. Drag the gray scroll bar in the middle of the screen to the top.
2. Click on 3½ Floppy (A)
3. Right click the file name junk.doc
3. The file name will become highlighted. Type junk2.doc

COPY A FILE FROM A FLOPPY TO THE HARD DRIVE

1. Use the scroll bar in the middle of the screen to move up until you see 3½ Floppy (A)
2. Click 3½ Floppy (A)
3. Right-click the name of the file junk.doc
4. Click Copy.
5. Scroll back down to the Windows directory.
6. Right-click the name of the Windows directory and select Paste.
7. Click the View menu, then Refresh so the file list will be updated.
8. Scroll over and look for junk2.wri
9. Click File, Close to close Explorer.

FIND A FILE

1. Click the Start button on the lower left of the screen.
2. Click Find, then Files or Folders.
3. Type `junk` and press the Enter key.
4. Wait a minute as the computer looks for the file.

DELETE A FILE

1. Right-click Start; then Explore.
2. Drag gray scroll bar in the middle of the screen to the top.
3. Click on 3½ Floppy (A)
4. Click the name of the file junk2.doc
5. Click the File menu, then Delete. (Or press the Delete key.)
6. Click OK.

RECOVER A DELETED FILE

1. Follow the above procedure to delete the file junk.doc from the c:\Windows directory.
2. Right-click an open area of the taskbar along the bottom of the screen.
3. Click Minimize All Windows.
4. Right-click the Recycle Bin.
5. Click Open.
6. Right-click the file name junk.doc
7. Click Restore. The file will return to the directory it was deleted from.

G. WINDOWS 95 ONLINE HELP

1. Click the Start button, then Help.
2. This opens the Windows 95 help function.
3. Click the Contents tab once.
4. Click Windows Tour, then Display.
5. This is a ten-minute guided tour of common functions such as starting a program, finding files, or switching between two programs.

II. Problem-Solving

- Figure out what devices the cables in the back of your case connect to. If they were disconnected, could you put them back in again? (Don't try to disconnect them unless the computer is turned off!)
- In Windows 3.1, create a program group (in Windows 95, a folder), name it "Internet" and put shortcuts to Netscape or Explorer into it.

III. Thought and Discussion

- Five years from now computers will probably be able to recognize speech or talk back to us. How might that change medical practice?
- Tools extend the capacity of people in various ways; for example, a shovel extends our reach and leverage. How does a computer extend our capacity?
- Compare the process of learning to start an IV, learning to speak a language, and learning to use a computer.
- Imagine that you are using a telephone-style Internet connection to speak to a help desk. At the end of the conversation your screen shows this message: "If you want to speak to a real person, click here." Does this mean that the computer you were speaking with is "intelligent?"

Readings From the Net

(Links available at http://NewWindPub.com/workbook)

Windows

Introduction to Windows	http://www.microsoft.com/windows/software/reskit.htm	Excellent short how-to for basic tasks in Windows 3.1
Microsoft	http://www.microsoft.com	Extensive documentation.
Windows 95	http://www.cs.umb.edu/~alilley/win.html	Very specific and detailed.
Question Answer Information Depot	http://www.kingsoft.com/qaid	Easy to read, well-organized introductions, tips, troubleshooting.

Chapter 3: Browsers and the Web

But it is not the visions but the activity which makes you happy, and the joy and glory of the flyer is the flight itself.

Isak Dineson, Out of Africa

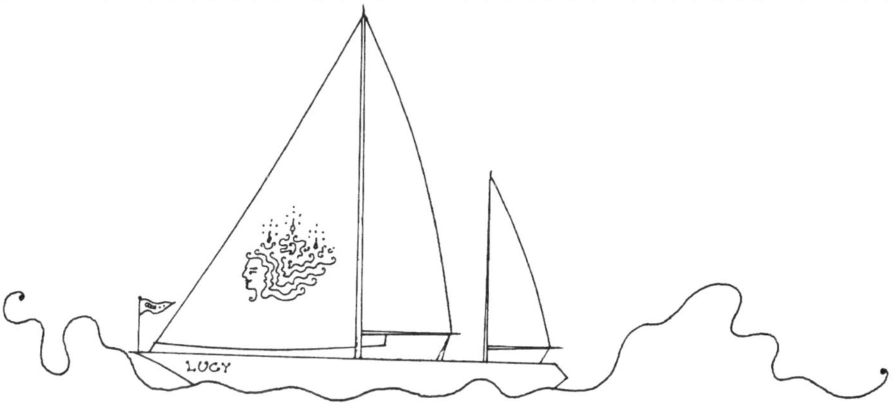

IN THIS CHAPTER

bandwidth
browser
client
configuration
download
helper application
Microsoft Explorer
modem
Netscape Navigator
server
service provider
shell account
UNIX

Browsers and Other Animals

The main purpose of an Internet browser is to display Web pages, although it can do much more. Approximately eighty percent of people connected to the Web use the browser called Netscape Navigator, and most of the remaining twenty percent use Microsoft Explorer. (Don't confuse Internet Explorer with Microsoft's file manager, also called Explorer.) Popular online services (America Online, Compuserve, Prodigy) include Web browsers with their software. In addition, Microsoft Explorer can be used with America Online, and Netscape Navigator with Compuserve or Prodigy.

Nothing in the world changes as fast as Web browsers. Navigator, only a few years old, is already in its fourth major version. (This chapter describes both version 3, which many people are using, and version 4, Communicator, which is in a preview release at the time of writing.) You can expect browsers to add significant new features at least once a year for the next few years.

Using an older version of most computer programs will not affect your work. Browsers, on the other hand, work with ever-changing Web sites. Browsers age so fast that even fruit flies have a hard time keeping up. If the one you are using is more than a couple of years old, chances are it is missing some essential functions. Older browsers can't handle such things as forms, Java, or tables, not to mention video, encryption, or email directories. The Internet is becoming so important that upcoming versions of Navigator and Explorer are aiming to become the gateway to all your programs and files.

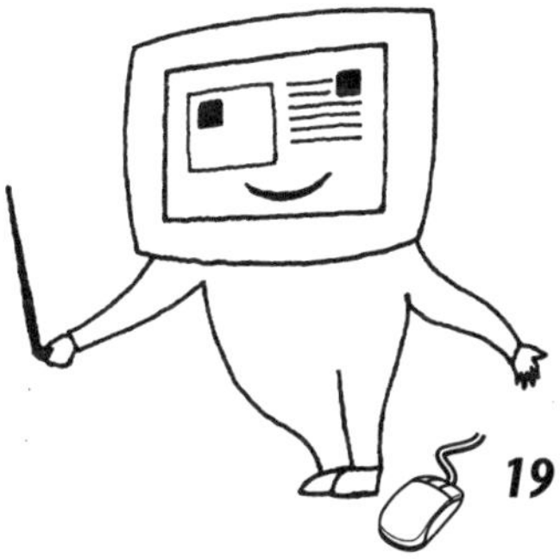

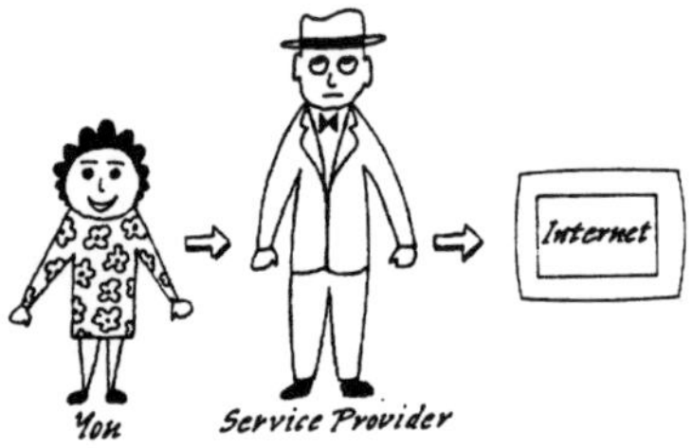

Connecting to the Internet

Even if the computer you are using in school or at work is already connected to the Internet, you may need to set up a computer at home. What will you need to access the Internet?

1. computer with a modem
2. service provider or online service
3. browser

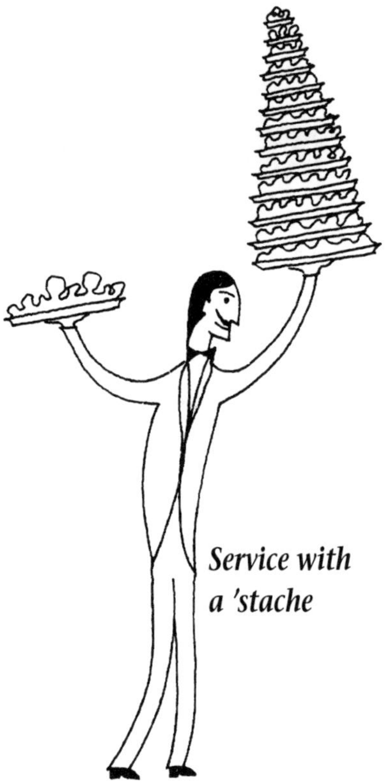

Service with a 'stache

A modem is standard equipment on most new computers. The modem has a jack that a telephone cord plugs into; the other end plugs into your phone jack in the wall. When you dial your service provider, you will hear a few seconds of noise as it connects to your service provider's modem. This is called handshaking, although handscreeching might be more apt.

The hardest part is setting up the operating system software in your computer so that it can connect to the Internet. The most common type of connection is called SLIP or PPP. (An older kind of connection, used with Unix computers, is called a shell account.) Configuring a computer so that it will work requires going through several steps (in Windows 95) or installing a special program (called Trumpet Winsock) in Windows 3.1. You will have to type in IP addresses, mail server names, gateway names, and other odd parameters and info-flotsam. I recommend getting expert help, either from a friend who has done it before or from a technician with the service provider.

Service Provider

Although you can plug your modem into the telephone jack in the wall, that isn't sufficient for connecting to the Internet, any more than plugging your TV cable into a jack in the wall will give you cable TV. An Internet connection is a service which you pay for, usually with a monthly fee, to an Internet service provider. (Online services are one type of provider.) The easiest way to find a provider is to look in the phone book under Internet.

> **Service Provider**
>
> A company that sells access to the Internet.

The most important question to ask any provider of computer software, hardware, or service is what kind of help they offer when things go wrong. This is especially true of companies which offer connections to the Internet. Ask them what hours and days a technical person can be reached by phone; whether they have a Web site with documentation; whether they have paper handouts; and so on. They should give you all the time you need. If they rush you, or if they are difficult to reach by telephone, or if you feel at all confused when talking to them, go elsewhere.

Questions to ask a Service Provider

You may not understand all these points right now. Look in the Glossary for unfamiliar words.

- Do they have different kinds of service for individuals, non-profit, and companies? (This is common.)
- Is space for a personal Web site included? (It should be.) If so, does their Web server process forms? Do they have secure credit card interactions? Do they provide log file reports? Is the traffic for your Web site metered?
- How many email addresses are included? (Usually one or two.)
- What is the top speed of connection? (It should be no less than 28.8 kbps, kilobits per second)
- Is this shell access, SLIP, or PPP? (Should be SLIP/PPP.)
- Do they include Domain Name registration? (You may want this later, if you set up a Web site with them.)
- Do they provide any software, such as a browser? (This will save you time in the beginning.)
- What kind of help is available, and during what hours? (Telephone, email, walk-in?)

Beyond Browsing: FTP, Telnet, Gopher, Email

On the Internet you can do more than browse for Web pages: you can send email, download programs, read bulletin boards, run distant computers. In the past, each function required a separate program (often referred to as a "client,") and even today the bookstores are full of swollen texts explaining the intricacies of strange programs like Pico and Tin (Rin-Tin?). But leave the ten-pound tomes for someone else: software that comes with many online services (e.g. America Online, Compuserve, Prodigy, Netcom) has easy-to-use components for each of these different functions.

The current version of Netscape (Communicator) is a good example. It is really many programs in one:

- Web browser
- email program
- newsgroup reader
- telnet program
- Web page editor
- calendar and task organizer
- conferencing, whiteboard and chat program

Email is explained in Chapter 5, and the use of newsgroup readers in Chapter 14.

A Web server sends pages to your browser.

A browser such as Navigator or Explorer is called a client program because it makes requests for Web pages. The computers that answer these requests are called Web servers: they are the storehouses of the pages that are sent to your screen. Web servers provide Web pages; email servers store and deliver email messages; newsgroup servers store newsgroup messages; file servers store files; and so on.

If you look at Appendix C, you will find that you can download programs for email, newsgroups, ftp, audio, video, animation, multimedia, news broadcasting, and a few other possibilities. Do you need all these in order to browse the Web?

Helper Application

A program that runs alongside your browser to extend its capabilities.

Not yet. Most of the Web is still text and pictures. Although browsers soon will have video and audio built into them, these files are still impractical to send at current modem speeds. Plug-ins or helper applications are programs that work with different kinds of files, such as video. Although you can certainly download these programs, the fundamental way that information is exchanged on the Web today is through text and graphics.

EXERCISES

Each lettered exercise is independent.
(Links available at http://NewWindPub.com/workbook)

I. Guided Practice

A. EMAIL A WEB PAGE TO YOURSELF

Send a Web page using the email function directly from Netscape. This sends the html codes along with the content of the page.

1. Start Netscape or Explorer.
2. Go to any page, or use the home page.
3. Click File, Mail Document. (Netscape 4: File, Send Page; Explorer: File, Send To.)
4. Type in your email address.
5. Click the Send button, or (in the email window) File, Send Now.
6. Wait for the message window to disappear, which indicates that the message has been sent.

B. COPY THE CONTENTS OF A WEB PAGE INTO AN EMAIL MESSAGE.

1. Start Netscape or Explorer.
2. Go to any page, or use the home page.
3. Click Edit, Select All.
4. Click Edit, Copy.
5. Click File, New Mail Message. (Netscape 4: Click Communicator, Messenger Mailbox. Then click the New Message button; Explorer: File, New Message.)
6. Type in your email address.
7. Tab until the cursor is in the main text area, or click anywhere in that text area.
8. Click Edit, Paste.
9. Click the Send button, or (in the email window) File, Send Now.
10. Wait for the message window to disappear.

C. ADD A BOOKMARK TO A PAGE

1. Start Netscape or Explorer.
2. Go to any page, or use the home page.
3. Click Bookmarks, Add Bookmark. (Explorer: Favorites, Add to Favorites.)
4. Click Bookmarks again.
5. Look for the title of your page at the bottom of the list.

D. SAVE A WEB PAGE TO THE HARD DRIVE

Save a Web page as a file to your hard drive, then open the page from the hard drive.

1. Start Netscape or Explorer.
2. Go to any page, or use the home page.
3. Click File, Save As. (Explorer: File, Save as File.)
4. Type in `junk.htm`
5. Click Save.
6. Click File, Open File (Netscape 4: File, Open Page; Explorer: File, Open, Browse)
7. Click the file name junk.htm, then on Open. (Netscape 4: Click Choose File, junk.htm, Open, Open.)
8. Look at the Location bar to double-check where the page came from. It should show the c: drive.

E. CHECK LENGTH OF A PAGE BEFORE PRINTING

1. Start Netscape. (Not available in Explorer.)
2. Go to http://www.gen.emory.edu/MEDWEB
3. Click Keyword Index.
4. Under Alternative Medicine, click By subcategory.
5. Click ALL SITES. This is a long document.
6. To see how many pages it will be if printed, click the File menu, then Print Preview.
7. When the page is showing and the mouse pointer is the shape of a magnifying glass, click anywhere on the lower left of the page to zoom in.
8. You will see "Page 1 of ..."
9. Or to count the pages, click the Next Page button at the top of the screen repeatedly.
10. Click Close to exit the print preview.

II. Problem-Solving

- Change the way Netscape displays links to bright red.
- Change the home page of your browser to point to another Web page.

III. Thought and Discussion

- Compare the organization of the Web, the human brain, and the Library of Congress.
- What is different about communicating face to face, by letter, by telephone, by email, or by sign language?

Readings From the Net

(Links available at http://NewWindPub.com/workbook)

The World Wide Web

Atlas to the World Wide Web	http://www.rhythm.com/~bpowell/Atlas/toc.htm	Combination text and directory (over 800 sites). Lots of graphics, links and other content.
Browser Watch	http://browserwatch.iworld.com	News, info, the latest on browsers. Technical.
The Help Web	http://www.imagescape.com/helpweb	Very friendly, with small collections of pointers on topics such as email, ftp, Web.
Netizens: An Anthology	http://www.columbia.edu/~rh120	Scholarly, upbeat, high-tech volume on the Net, emphasizing political and philosophical issues.
Netscape home page	http://home.netscape.com	More than just info about the program.
Que Bookshelf	http://www.mcp.com/que/bookshelf	Go to "Special Edition using Netscape 3" This is the entire thousand-page book!
The Virtual Community	http://www.well.com/www/hlr/vcbook	The complete text of the book by Howard Rheingold. California tone and perspective.

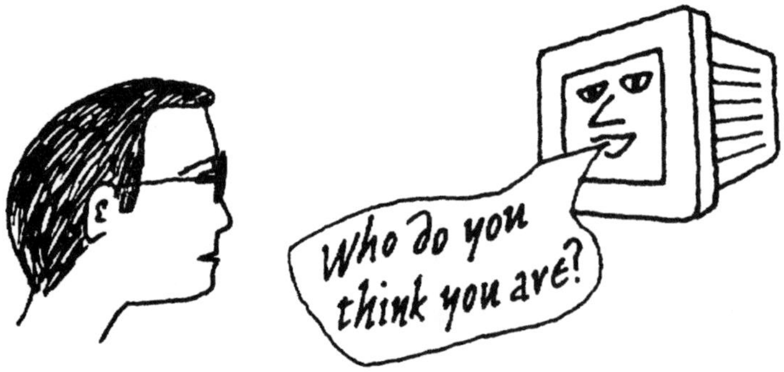

Chapter 4: Anatomy of a Website

Good design is simple, bold, and direct.
Kevin Mullet and *Darrell Sano*,
Designing Visual Interfaces

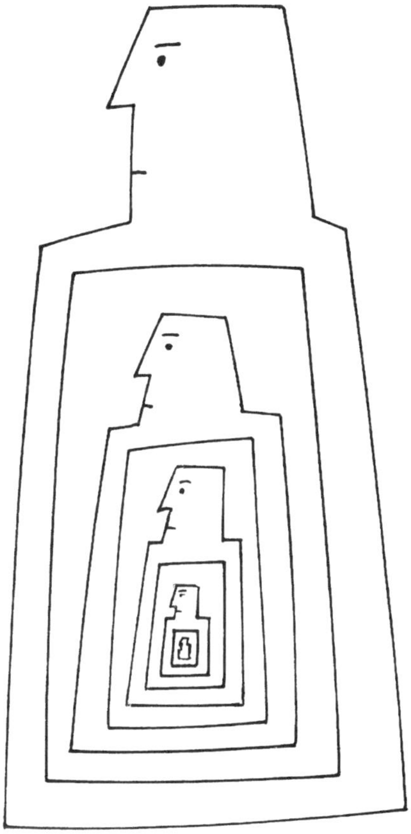

IN THIS CHAPTER

button bar
chat
cookie
domain name
encryption
frame
FTP
gopher
host
HTML
HTTP
imagemap
IP address
navigation bar
security
thumbnail graphic
VRML

A Web site is really a collection of documents in digital form. What will you find there? Text, pictures, sound clips, animation, even video. You get to a site by following a link from another Web page, or by typing the address into the location bar of your browser, as we did in Chapter 1.

Think of a Web site as a building. The home page of a Web site is the front door, so to speak, which leads to everything else you will find on the site. The building is organized into floors, and on each floor you find rooms.

Most commercial, educational, and government Web sites will have their own name, such as www.healthgate.com. Many individual sites will have the name of their provider, followed by the individual's name: www.somecompany.com/my_name/

Domain Name
The top-level name for an Internet site, such as mycompany.com

New domains 1997

.nom	personal
.firm	businesses or firms
.store	goods to purchase
.web	related to the WWW
.arts	cultural
.rec	recreation
.info	information services

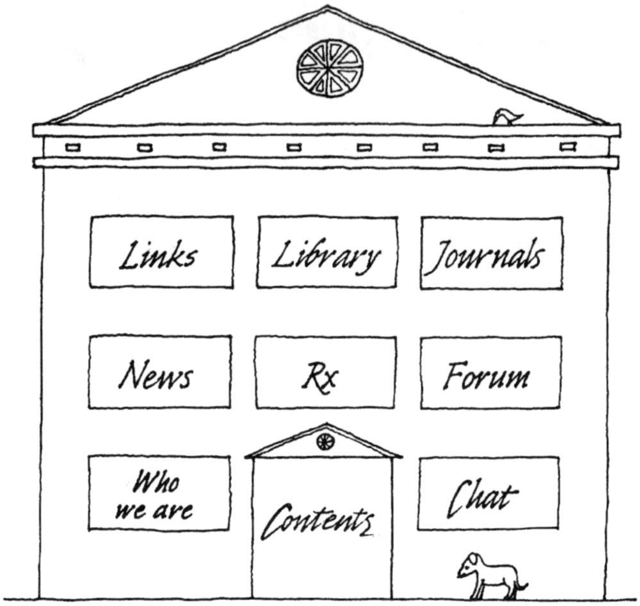

Common Home Page Information

On the home page you should be able to see a table of contents showing you where to find things, much as you expect to see a directory when you walk into a large building. If a site is organized well, the home page will give you a quick idea of what the site is for and what you will find on it.

The home page of most well-constructed sites will give you an introduction to the site, a table of contents, a search box, the name of the company or organization that put up the site, an email contact, and a copyright notice. Commercial sites will often have ugglesome advertisements (called banners), which may have moving text or animated images.

Often you will get to a site by following a link, but you will not land initially on the home page. Look around on the top or the bottom of the page for a link that says Home. Sometimes you will see a link that says Back or Top, or perhaps an icon of a house.

An Important Trick

If you land on a page but don't see any such links, here is a little-known trick for getting to the home page, from which you may find the page you want. This also works if you get a message back saying "Page not found."

Look at the address of the page in the location bar. ***Click to position the cursor to the right of the address, backspace to erase everything after the first single slash, and press the Enter key.***

For example, if you tried to go to a page whose address is:
http://vh.radiology.uiowa.edu/Providers/ClinRef/FPHandbook/
FPContents.html
and you didn't know what site it belonged to, or the page had moved, then erase everything after the word com so it reads:
http://vh.radiology.uiowa.edu
and press the Enter key. This will take you to the home page.

Frames

On some sites you see a rectangular area, often along the left of the screen, that has its own scroll bar. When you move from page to page on the site, this area remains the same. This is called a frame. Frames are used to show links to the main areas of a site, so that you will always be able to see the links and get to those areas.

A page may have two or more frames, each with its own information. To see an extensive use of frames, go to Dr. Schueler's On-line Medical Glossary (http://www.drschueler.com/glossary/glossary.htm).

Button Bar and Navigation Bar

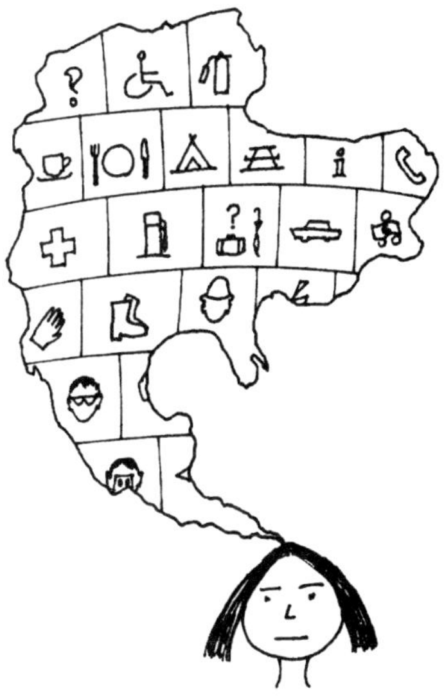

Imagemap?

Another way to do the same thing is to put a standard set of links to the main areas at the top or bottom of each page on a site. This is called a button bar because the links often look like buttons you push on a stereo, or a navigation bar, because the buttons are links to other parts of the site.

A common icon in button bars is an arrow pointing to the left, which takes you back to the previous page; an arrow pointing up which takes you to a higher level; or an arrow pointing right which takes you to the next page.

Programs also have rows of buttons for the more common functions available in that program. For example Netscape has Back, Forward, and Home buttons.

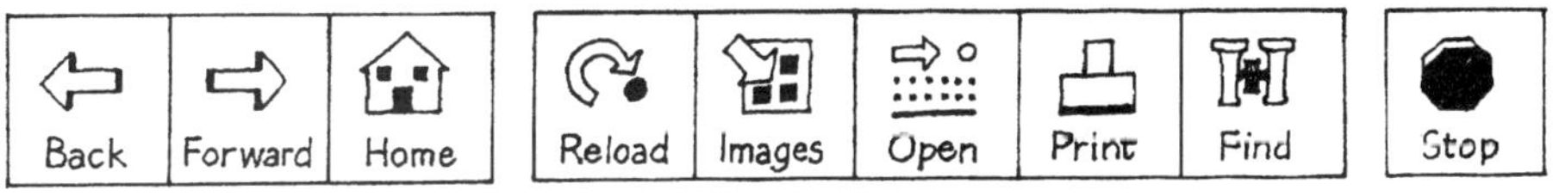

Pictures To Go

A button bar is one example of how an image can be a link to something else. In general, pictures that do this are called imagemaps. The home page for a site may use a large picture as an imagemap that you use to jump to different parts of the site. Take a look at the Web site for the Centers for Disease Control (http://www.cdc.gov) to see how a large imagemap can be used as a pictorial table of contents.

Most sites that use pictures as links will still have text links along the bottom of the page.

Thumbnail

A small version of a picture.

Thumbnails

Because larger pictures can take a long time to transfer at current modem speeds, often you will see a tiny version of a picture on a Web page, called a thumbnail, which links to the larger version. With the use of thumbnail graphics a Web designer can include several pictures on a page, and yet the page will still download quickly. To see the larger picture, double-click the thumbnail version.

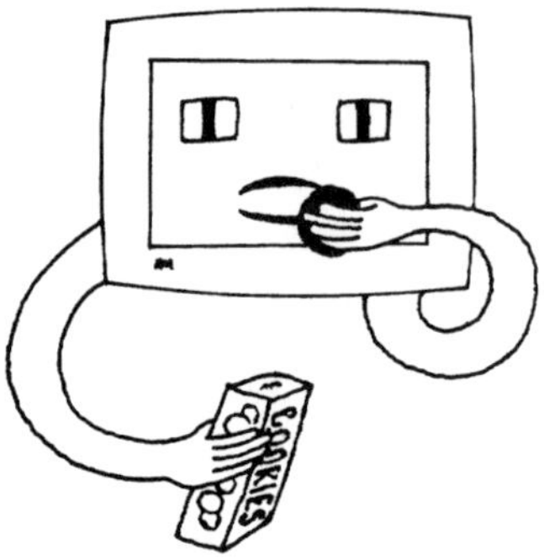

Cookies and other Transactions

A cookie is a piece of information that the site sends to your computer, which can be used to track information about your visit to the site. Browsers can be set to accept or reject cookies, or warn you when a cookie is being sent. Cookies are really one example of a more general phenomenon called transactions, when one machine or program sends information to another.

What's going on with cookies? When a Web page is sent to your browser, it is an isolated event, much like sending a letter. No connection is maintained between your computer and the server where the page came from, and the server won't "recognize" you the next time you request a page. But in some cases a cookie may be useful (such as when you want to move in and out of a password-protected site without entering the password every time) or when placing items into a virtual shopping cart as you move from page to page on a commercial site.

By using cookies, a site can save information about preferences, which enables a person to customize the view or function of certain pages. You decide how the pages are displayed or which links are visible, and the information is stored in the cookie file on your computer for the next time you visit that site.

A troubling problem with cookies is that they can enable Web sites to secretly collect information about you, for example the sites you have visited. See the discussion on privacy in Chapter 13.

HTTP

Skip this section if you're a techno-phobe. A protocol is a set of rules that lets different machines talk to each other, in the same way that diplomatic protocols let officials conduct meetings. If one computer is speaking French and another is speaking German, they won't be able to communicate.

Protocol

The rules that two computers use to exchange information.

The protocol for the World Wide Web is called hypertext transport protocol (HTTP). HTTP governs what kind of information can be included on a Web page, how it is sent, and anything that goes with the Web page, such as a picture or a chunk of program. Other protocols in use on the Internet are file transfer protocol (FTP), simple mail transport protocol (SMTP), gopher, or network news transport protocol (NNTP).

At a lower level than hypertext transport protocol, TCP/IP governs the basic way that all information is packaged, routed, and delivered, whether it be an email message, Web page, or video clip. Because it is a reliable and efficient protocol, and a worldwide standard, TCP/IP is increasingly being used within healthcare and business organizations as well as over the Internet.

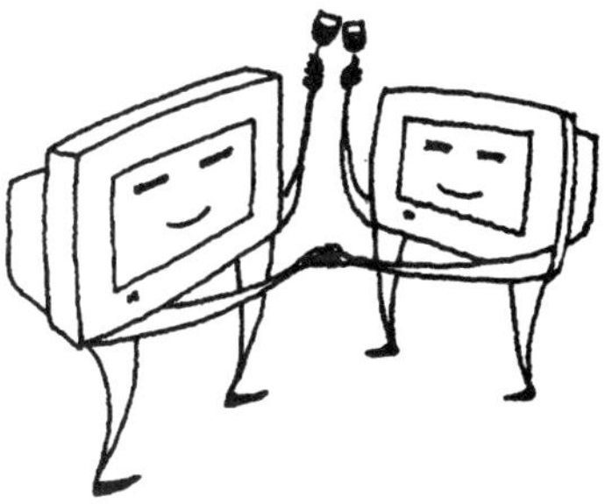

Franco-Germanic protocol

HTML

For a document to transfer using hypertext transport protocol, it must be formatted using HTML, the hypertext markup language. This language is a set of codes or symbols that a browser uses to format the page with such design elements as bold or centered text, boxes, tables, or imagemaps.

In the past, if you wanted to create a Web page, you needed to learn HTML codes, which was tantamount to programming. That's no longer true. Netscape will send email as HTML, and most word processors now give you the choice of saving a document as a Web page. These days you do not have to learn programming to create a Web page!

> HTML
>
> hypertext markup language

Forms

As a medical professional you probably use admission and discharge forms, flow sheets, order entry forms. A form on the computer is used for similar purposes, but instead of writing the information you type it into a text box.

A form may have check boxes, radio buttons, and drop-down lists in addition to text boxes. These give you different ways of making choices.

Security

Forms are a convenient way to gather information. How do you know that the information you type into a form, such as your social security number or a credit card number, isn't being intercepted by someone in its journey across the Internet?

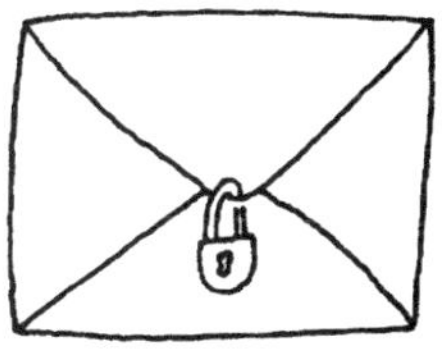

> *Encryption*
>
> To put a message into secret code so it can't be intercepted.

The simple answer is that you don't. Protocols have been developed (SSL and SHTTP) to encrypt information so that it can only be decoded by an authorized computer, but these methods are barely keeping up with crackers and other unscrupulous geeks who are trying to break encryption codes. Let the browser beware.

Netscape 3.0 shows a key at the bottom right of the screen which is broken if the site is not secure. Netscape 4 has a separate window for security information about a site. As a general rule, if you are not sure whether sending some information (such as a credit card number) is safe, don't do it.

Tables

A table divides a page into rows and columns, like this:

	column 2	column 3	column 4
row 2			
row 3			
row 4			

Tables are a very effective way to organize information (see Chapter 17, Creating Information). They can also be used in Web pages to place text into columns, or to create a margin where small pictures or samples of text can be placed.

Animation

Animation means pictures which move. Animation is a common (and often annoying) aspect of the Web. One type of moving picture (in a picture format called gif) does not need any special software, and can be created with simple programs by stringing pictures together the way you made flip cards as a kid. Other, more spiffy animations use special software such as Shockwave; to see these your browser needs an add-on program called a plug-in to see the animation.

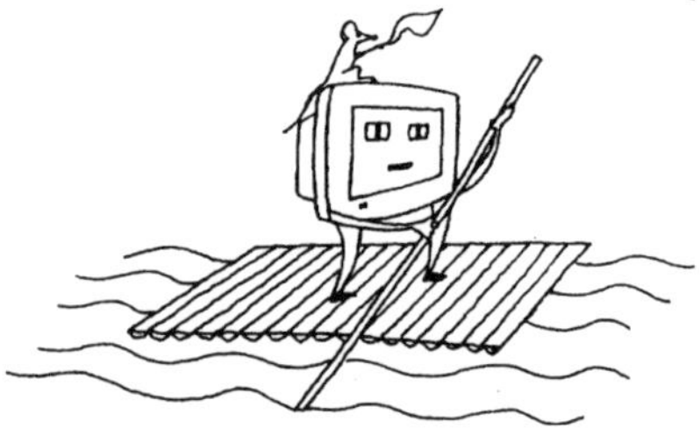

Streaming video

Video

During 1997 the worlds of television and the Internet moved closer together. A Web page can display video images, but these images are still relatively rare on the Net because they take so long to download at today's modem speeds. MPEG (Moving Picture Experts Group) is the standard for storing and transmitting video images. There are several different standards, one used for digital video disks (DVD), another for high definition television (HDTV), and another for Internet images (MPEG). The next version, MPEG-4, is supposed to set the standard for speech synthesis, fractal images, and computer visualization.

Because modem speeds are still relatively slow compared to the size of video and sound files, and to make their transmission more efficient, a new method for transmitting them has been developed, called streaming. Past methods required the whole file to be sent before it could be displayed. Streaming allows the video to be seen, or the sound to be heard, as the file arrives.

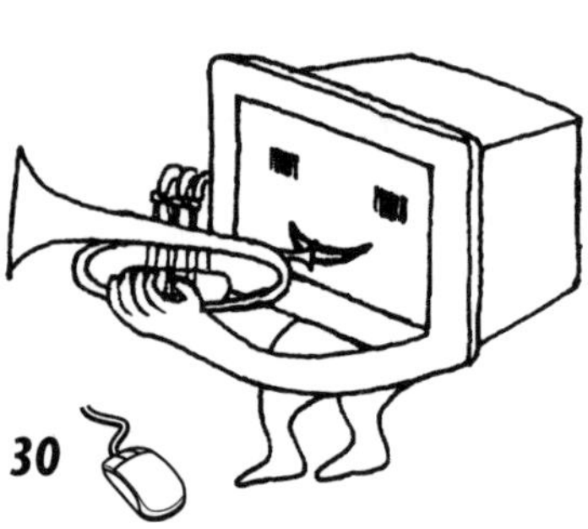

Sounds and Music

As with video, sound must be stored and transmitted in a digital form for use on the Internet. In addition to having a browser or application that can play the sounds, your computer must have speakers and a sound card. Most computers purchased since 1996 will have these.

Animation, sound and video may be included within a Web page and start as soon as the page appears, or they may be included as links or thumbnails that you click to activate.

Channels

Everyone has a general idea of what a "channel" is, based on experience with television channels. Whether there are three or three hundred, each channel transmits a particular group of shows and information. Special-interest channels may be limited to shows on sports, science-fiction, or news.

Internet companies are actively developing technologies that will send you "channels" of information in much the same way. Pointcast was one of the first, but many more are now involved. Channel technology on the Internet begins to blur the distinction between browsing and viewing; information may be "pushed" to a computer screen along a specific channel, rather than waiting on a Web site for a person to browse and find it.

Three-Dimensional Images

A three-dimensional image or scene on a computer is called virtual reality. VRML (Virtual Reality Markup Language) is used to create sites called rooms or worlds. Unlike regular images, you can go behind or inside of a VRML object.

Virtual
Simulated, not real.

VRML may have important uses in medicine and health care, especially for training. Imagine being able to maneuver through three-dimensional images of the heart, lungs, kidneys, and brain! Or set up a training site for "virtual" surgery, using VRML patients. Howard Rheingold says in *Virtual Reality* that "the power to create experience is also the power to redefine such basic concepts as identity, community, and reality."

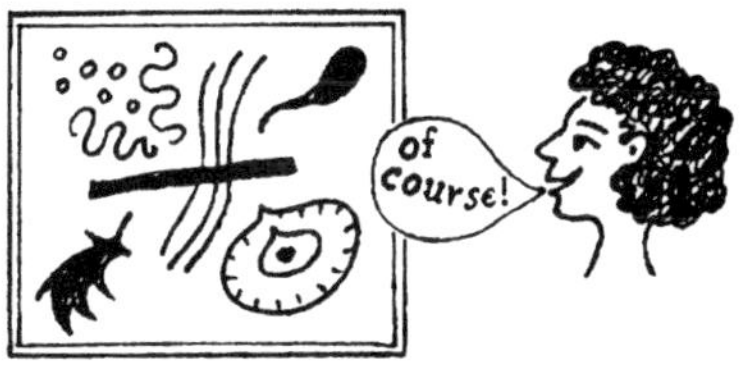

In 1945 Vannevar Bush, the first to realize the ability of hypertext as an extension of a person's knowledge, wrote: "In the next generation, technical advance and basic scientific discovery will be inseparable." With the progress of computers, anything you can imagine related to information is likely to come to pass, even within a generation. Hopefully this chapter has whetted your appetite for more of the virtual widgets hitting the shelves every day. So pick an avatar, find your center of gravity, and hang on: we're in for an exciting ride.

EXERCISES

Each lettered exercise is independent.
(Links available at http://NewWindPub.com/workbook)

I. *Guided Practice*

A. EXPLORE A PATIENT-ORIENTED WEB SITE

Learn about frames, tables, button bars, forms, forums, and email links from a site devoted to patient education.

1. Start Netscape or Explorer..
2. Go to http://medhlp.netusa.net
3. Along the top is the button bar, in its own frame. Scroll down the page. Note that the MedHelp button bar stays visible.
4. Note the table format of the page.
5. Click About in the MedHelp button bar.
6. Click Our Advisory Board. Note that the link is internal, to a point further down on the same page.
7. Click the Back button. Note that this returns you to the top of the same page.

MAILTO: LINK

A mailto link looks like a hypertext link, but instead of jumping to a page, Netscape starts up its email program with a person's address already entered.

1. Click MedHelp in the MedHelp button bar to return to their home page.
2. Scroll down to the bottom of the page.
3. Click e-mail: staff@medhelp.org
4. This starts up the Netscape email program with a message addressed to staff@medhelp.org
5. In the email window, click File, Close to cancel the message.

FORUM

A forum is a way for people to communicate together. This one is like Usenet, with questions and answers. It uses a form.

1. Click Forums and Messages in the MedHelp button bar.
2. Click The MedHelp General Forum.
3. Click the first link that has a date by it.
4. Click Follow Ups. This takes you further down on the same page. If anyone has answered the note, a link will be here.
5. Scroll down the page to the area that says Post a Follow Up. Here is a form that you would fill out to post a reply to the note you are reading.
6. Use the Back button to return to the list of messages.
7. Click any message where the author is listed as Med Help International.
8. This is a reply posted by the moderators of the Web site itself to a patient question.

B. WEB-BASED CHAT

Chat is like a conference call. It is a means for people to type (or talk) in "real time." Instead of posting a message and waiting (as with a forum) you see the messages as they occur.

1. Start Netscape or Explorer.
2. Go to http://www.nursingnet.com/chat
3. Click the text box, type in a name, and press the Enter key (or click the Enter button.)
4. If a window pops up "Security Information," press the Enter key.
5. You may get this message: "The name you selected is already taken. Please select another name." If so, use the Back button, then try another name.
6. Note which chat area you are in.
7. Click in the text box to the right of "Your Message..." and type in a message.
8. Click Post. It should appear in the lower part of the screen.
9. Click the text box next to the "Choose Chat Topic..." line and click another topic.
10. Click Go To. This puts you into a different "room."
11. Click the Netscape Back button to return to the Welcome page. Scroll down and click Return to the Nursing Resource Home page. (or go to http://www.nursingnet.com).
12. Take a look around. This is a good site for general nursing resources.

C. IMAGEMAPS AND THUMBNAIL IMAGES

Explore images that have hypertext links built into them (imagemaps) and tiny previews of images (thumbnails).

1. Start Netscape or Explorer.
2. Go to http://vh.radiology.uiowa.edu
3. This page will take a minute to load.

4. Move the cursor over the image. Note that when it passes over the areas "Welcome..." "For Patients" etc. it becomes a pointing hand.
5. Click For Healthcare Providers.
6. Click Multimedia Textbooks.
7. Click Pediatric Airway Disease.
8. Click the name of either author to see a photo and short biographical profile.
9. Click the Back button.
10. Scroll down and click the Anatomy section.
11. Note the small "thumbnail" images in the text.
12. Click an image to see an enlarged, annotated version.
13. Click the Back button to the chapter outline.
14. Click Croup Syndromes.
15. The first image is a link to a movie that is 1.6 megabytes. If you are at a computer with a fast network, you can click this. With a modem the movie will take too long to download.
16. Click Sound. If your computer has speakers, this will play the sound of an infant with croup.

D. COMMERCIAL SITE

This demonstrates a site with advertising banners, areas that are free versus those which require registration, and a preview of MEDLINE.

1. Start Netscape or Explorer.
2. Go to http://www.healthgate.com
3. Note the table of contents along a frame on the left.
4. Position the mouse pointer on the vertical bar separating the two frames. Click the bar and drag it a little to the right.
5. Click Free Pages.
6. Click Healthy Living.
7. Note the advertising banner at the top of the page. If you click it you will go to the site that is advertised.
8. Scroll down and click a thumbnail image, which links to a specific area.

MEDLINE

1. Click HealthGate Home on the HealthGate list along the left.
2. Click Search Medline.
3. Click in the box to the right of "Enter Search Terms," type in `gastritis`, and click Retrieve Documents.
4. Wait a minute or two.
5. Scroll down to see your results.
6. Click a title to see the abstract. Chapter 9 covers MEDLINE in depth.

REGISTRATION AREA

1. Click MedGate on the list along the left.
2. Click Drug Information Handbook.
3. Note that you get a window that says "Enter Username and Password..."
4. To see this resource you must be registered with HealthGate. Click Cancel.

II. Problem-Solving

- Look up the entry for malignant mesothelioma on Dr. Schueler's On-Line Medical Glossary (http://www.drschueler.com/glossary/glossary.htm).
- Look up today's medical news on Doctor's Guide (http://www.pslgroup.com/mednews.htm).

III. Thought and Discussion

- How can you quickly judge a Web site's worth?
- Is the Web a public resource, like a library, that should have free access?
- What might be the effect on society of the increasing amount of incorrect information being put on the Web? Should there be oversight or editorial control over all sites with medical information?

Readings From the Net

(Links available at http://NewWindPub.com/workbook)

The World Wide Web (more readings)

Entering the World Wide Web	http://www.hcc.hawaii.edu/guide/www.guide.html	From 1993; lots of pics.
Exploring the World Wide Web	http://www.gactr.uga.edu/Exploring/toc.html	Friendly, quick intros.
Internet Tutorial	http://www.msn.com/tutorial/default.html	Intro., surfing, advanced.
Web Reference	http://webreference.com	Select "Beginner Links."

Chapter 5: Electronic Mail

How can I know what I think till I see what I say?
Lewis Carroll, Alice in Wonderland

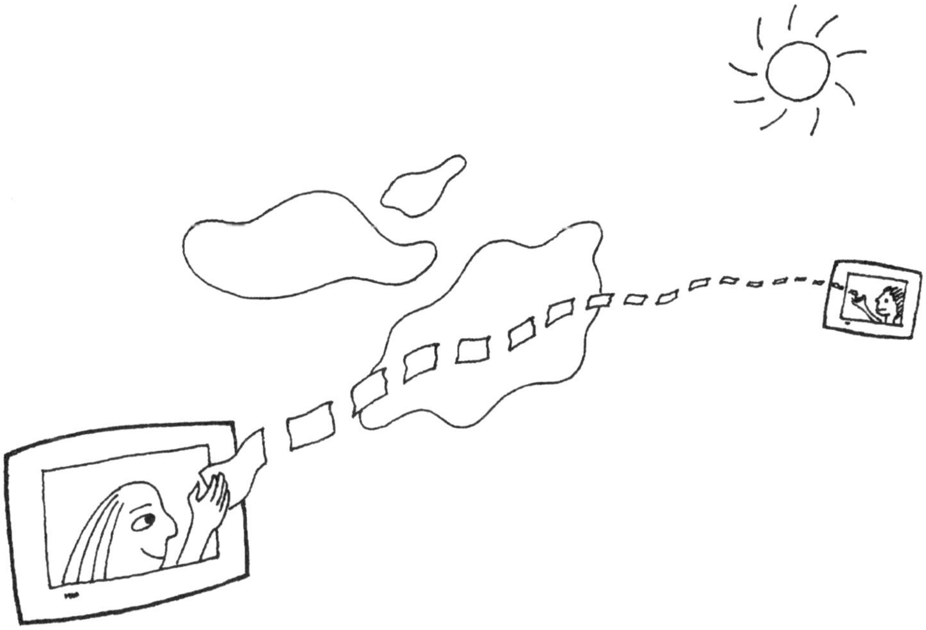

IN THIS CHAPTER

addressbook
alias
attachment
Bcc
Cc
email
filter
font
header
hosts
mailbox
MIME
Post Office Protocol
reply to all
return address
return receipt
signature
spell checker
subject line
trash

Electronic mail is the most widely used form of communication on the Internet. It's indispensable; in a few years every dunderhead will be using it. Although Internet technology is moving rapidly ahead with sound, video, animation and many other things, email will still be essential twenty years from now. Learning it is well worth the effort.

In concept, email is just like postal mail. Using an email program, you type a message and send it to the electronic address of another person. The message usually arrives in that person's electronic mailbox in a minute or two. After she checks for her mail and reads the message, she can respond to you, forward the note to another person, print it, or save it in an electronic folder.

Email is used widely on the Internet for many different kinds of communication. In addition to sending a note to one person, you can send a message to multiple people at once; post notes on the public bulletin board system known as the Usenet; or take part in group discussions via a mailing list. You can also attach a file to a message, such as a word processor document or a graphic picture. Email can even be linked to voice mail and pagers!

You must type an email address correctly, or it will bounce back to you.

Addresses

When you get an Internet account, you normally get an email box and one or more addresses as well. Other people use this address to send you email.

All email addresses are similar; they are in the form name@computer. The first part will usually be a person's name or initials. The second part gives the unique name for the computer where that person's mail is kept, in effect the electronic post office. This may be a business, university, hospital, or Internet provider.

You must type an email address exactly, or else it will return to you with an error message. It doesn't matter whether you capitalize the letters or not, but don't put any spaces in the address. To send a message to several people, put a comma and a space after each address, like this:
`person1@computer, person2@computer2, person3@computer3`

An addressbook can use an alias or a nickname instead of the email address; this means that when you type the alias, the program will substitute the actual email address before sending it. So you can send mail to John or Mary rather than m45xq@athena.verylongcompanyname.com

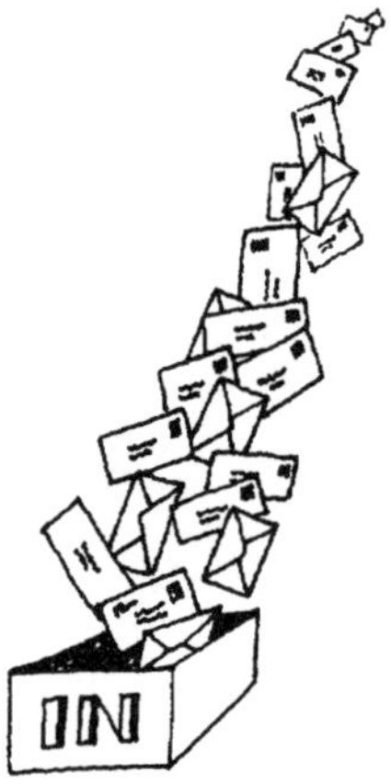

Where is the Mail?

When email is sent, it first goes to the computer called a mail server, run by an Internet service provider or institution. This computer is like a post office, except that it is open twenty-four hours a day. Messages stay in your personal email box on the mail server until you start your program, which then connects to the mail server and downloads the new mail to the inbox on your desktop computer. (You can also set up the program to wait for you to manually check for mail.) This whole process of storing mail on a server and then forwarding it to your email program is coordinated by the Post Office Protocol, or POP.

New Messages versus Saved Messages

Server
A computer that serves information upon request.

The mail server is not the same as your computer. Programs such as Eudora run on the computer at your desk. When you connect to the mail server, it sends any new messages to your desktop computer. The folders you create for your mail by using Eudora or Netscape are really files on your computer; these folders do not reside on the mail server.

Part of the confusion is that the word "inbox" is used both for a folder on your personal computer, and for the box on the mail server where messages are stored.

You will have a password for checking new mail, and because of this many people think that all their mail is "password protected." Not true. Even though you may enter a password for new messages that are waiting on the server for you, ***once you download mail to the inbox on your computer,* anybody who has access to your computer can read those messages.** If they are sensitive or private you must make sure that messages are saved in an area of the computer that only you can use, or in files that are protected by a password.

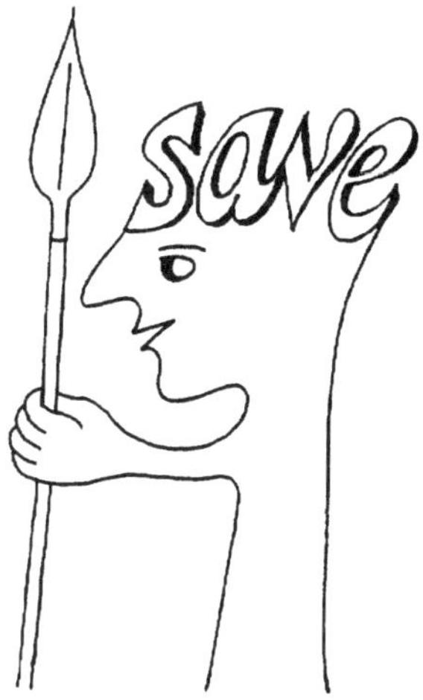

An older way of using email, which is still in use in many universities, keeps all mail and folders on the mail server. This has one major advantage: you can move from building to building, reading your mail from different computers, and always have access to your folders and saved mail. A newer way to work with email is to have all your folders kept on a Web server. You then read and send your mail through a Web page, and all the folders are stored on the Web server, rather than your desktop computer. Because messages are not stored on the desktop computer, there is no danger that other people will read them.

Subject Line

Every email message should have at least three items: the address where it is going, an entry in the subject line, and the message itself. You use the subject line to type a brief description of the message itself, such as *tomorrow's meeting* or *your proposal* or *hello out there.*

Use the subject line for a brief description of your message.

When you start your email program, if you have mail, you will see a list of messages. For each message you will see the subject as well as some other information. This lets you skim your messages at a glance to see which need to be read immediately.

Folders

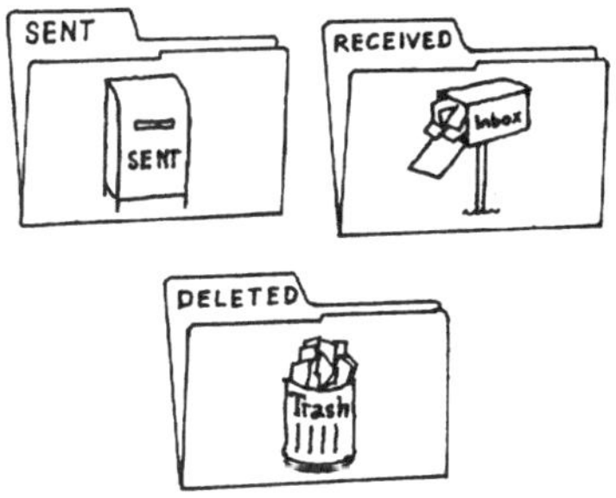

New messages typically arrive in a folder named the Inbox, but email programs let you create other electronic folders where you can move messages. After you read a message, you can delete it or move it to another folder.

One folder is commonly called trash. When you click the picture of a trash container or delete the message, it is moved to this folder. Until you close the program (or empty the Trash), you can go into the trash folder to retrieve any messages that have been put there.

Addressbook

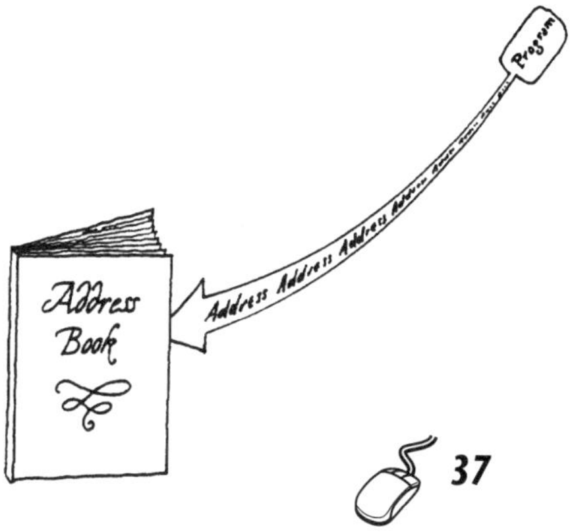

Most email programs give you an electronic addressbook where you can store names and addresses. When sending mail you can choose a name from your list, and the program will supply the address automatically. This prevents typing errors and saves you the trouble of remembering addresses.

Replying

When you are reading a message, you can reply to it by simply clicking on a Reply button. Usually, the original message will be automatically copied into the reply. This can be useful if you want to quote parts of it, or answer specific points, but you will help the other person if you delete all but the specific sections you are replying to. Otherwise you force her to read her own message all over again!

Be careful when replying!

You also have the choice of replying to everyone who got the original message. Be careful! Most of us are not familiar with the practice of sending a message to more than one person. If you reply to everyone who received the original, make sure that you are not saying something that is personal or confidential.

Cc: and Bcc:

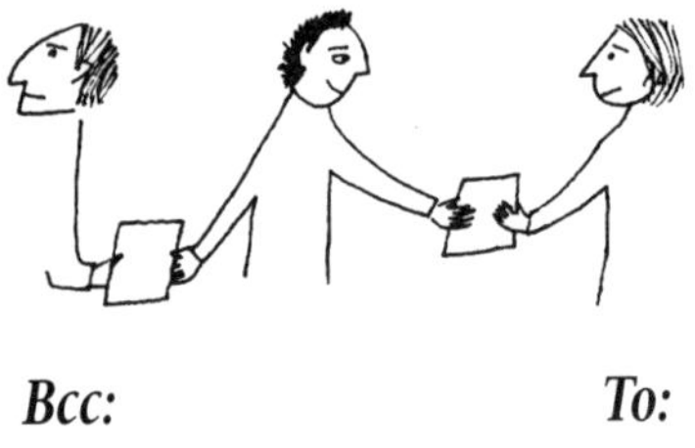

If you look at the bottom of a typed memo, it will often have a line which says Cc: followed by the names of several people. This means that each of them has received a "carbon copy" of the message. (These days most offices don't use carbon paper, but the name has stuck.) Email gives you the choice of putting an address in the Cc: line rather than the To: line, which can be useful if you want everyone to know who you are sending the "original" to and who is getting a "copy."

Bcc:

Blind Carbon Copy

The Bcc: line is a little trickier—and more useful. When you put someone's address in this line, his name will be hidden from all the others who receive it. (Bcc: stands for "Blind Carbon Copy".)

One use of the Bcc: function is to send a person a copy of a message so that others don't know he is getting it. You may also want to use the Bcc: line when you are sending a message to a large group, say fifty people. By hiding the addresses of all the other persons, you save each one the bother of scrolling through a large list of names to read the actual message. The first time you receive a one-line message with a hundred names at the top, you will understand how useful Bcc: is!

Attachments

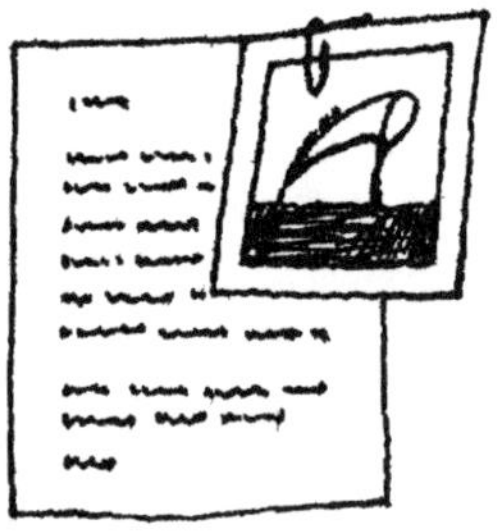

Email programs have the ability to attach other files to a message, for example a word processor document or a picture. When the other person receives the message, she then uses a word processor or graphics program to open and see the attachment. In this way different kinds of information can be sent using email.

An attachment must be changed into coded form to be sent with email, but not all email programs use the same standards for coding attachments. Just because your program can send it doesn't mean that the other person will be able to read it. The most common coding method is called MIME (Multipurpose Internet Mail Extensions). Macintosh computers use a protocol called BinHex, whereas Unix computers use one called Uuencode.

Signature

A person who answers a lot of mail may have a rubber stamp with her signature; rather than sign fifty letters, she will use the stamp. Email programs give you the ability to do something similar called an electronic signature, which is simply typed information that you want to be included at the bottom of each message that you send. A typical signature will have a person's full name, position, title or degree, and email address.

> *Signature*
>
> Lines that are automatically added to the bottom of your email messages.

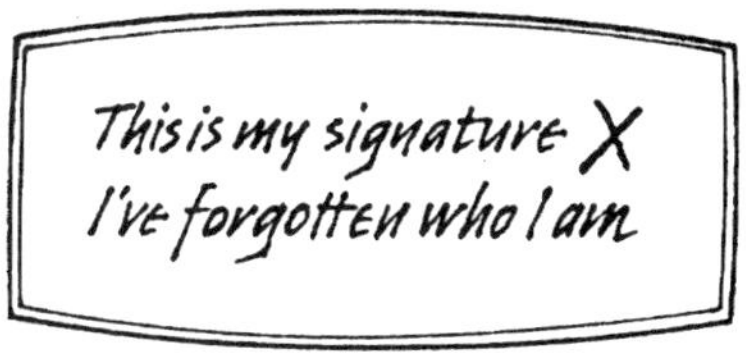

Filtering

Some programs include a function called a filter, which sorts your mail automatically. You can set up a filter to look for certain names or words in the address or message; for example, you can take all incoming mail from a friend and have it go into a folder that has her name. You can have all mail from a mailing list go to another folder. This is useful if you get a lot of email, or subscribe to several mailing lists. (See Chapter 14 for more about mailing lists.)

Return Receipt

When you take a letter to the post office you can request a return receipt, to make sure that the other person actually receives the letter. Email gives you an analogous function. With email programs you can request a return receipt that will automatically be sent to you when the other person opens your message. Note that it doesn't mean that the message has actually been read, but simply opened. Many people read email quickly, so don't get angry with someone because you received a return receipt but she didn't answer your specific questions.

Straight Text and Flavored Text

In the past, email messages were simple text. You couldn't make the words bold, or underlined, or color them green. In the newer versions of Eudora and Netscape you now have the ability to format the text with different sizes, colors, and fonts. Maybe this will slow down the onslaught of smileys and emoticons, those strange art forms intended to tell us whether a person is being ironic, humorous, or downright silly.

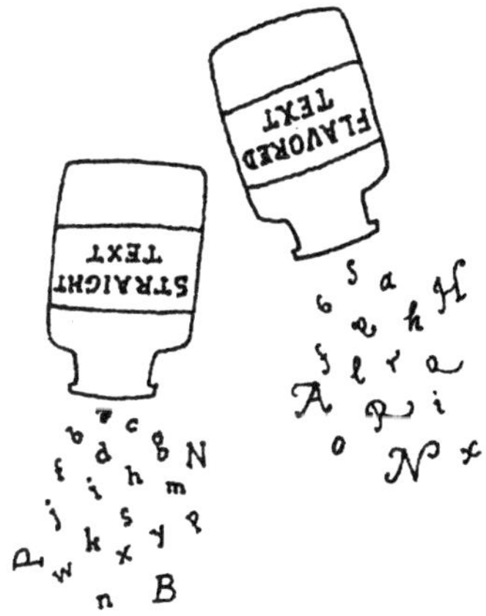

Free Email

It is possible to get an email box for free—even if you are homeless! Several Web sites offer this service (for example, see http://www.hotmail.com); and because public libraries now have computers with Web access, you don't need any money at all to get email. A service like this is financed by advertisements that you see on the screen when you send or receive email using their Web site.

Smiley

Face-drawings created by keyboard symbols, used to indicate emotions.

:)	happy
:-0	oops!
:- /	skeptical

Finding Email Addresses

Although there are many good directories of email addresses available on the Internet, there is no one place you can go to find a person's address. Some companies or commercial services do not give out addresses. See the exercises for a listing of places to go on the Internet to find an address.

A new protocol is now in use on the Internet that allows email programs to connect to a directory of email addresses. The Netscape 4 email addressbook, for example, has a box where you can choose to search a directory such as Switchboard to look for an address.

A Cautionary Word

Email is so much faster to compose and send than postal mail that everyone is a little giddy at first. You may find yourself dashing off quick notes and responses willy-nilly, without even looking at the screen. Remember that a thinko is just as likely as a typo, and may have worse consequences. It pays to read your words at least once before sending them skittering across cyberspace.

EXERCISES

Each lettered exercise is independent.
(Links available at http://NewWindPub.com/workbook)

I. *Guided Practice*

If you have a connection to the Internet, you can use Netscape or another email program to send and receive email. The exercises below cover Eudora and Netscape.

EUDORA (VERSION 2 OR 3)

The exercises are written for Eudora 3. Differences between Eudora 3 and Eudora 2 are noted under each section. Because one significant difference between Eudora 2 and 3 are the button bar icons, most exercises below use menu items instead.

A. SET UP EUDORA

You must first have access to the Internet on your computer, and an email account. The instructions below cover only the essentials of getting Eudora to the point where it will send and receive mail. There are many settings not discussed below.

1. Start Eudora.
2. Click the Tools, Options menu. (Eudora 2: Special, Settings)
3. Click Getting Started. (If you do not see "Getting Started," drag the scroll bar in this window to the top.)
4. *Pop account*: Enter your full login name and address, e.g. something like `john.doe@computer.school.edu` or `john.doe@pop3.mycompany.com`
5. The pop account is the crucial piece of information for receiving mail. Talk to your system administrator if you can't receive email.
6. Real name: Type your full name, e.g. John Doe.
7. Click Personal Info.
8. *Return address*: Type your email address, e.g. `john.doe@university.edu`
9. Click Hosts.
10. *SMTP*: Type the name of the email computer which sends mail. It will be something like smtp.university.edu or smtp.mycompany.com
11. This is the crucial piece of information for sending email. Talk to the system administrator if you can't send email.
12. These are the bare essentials. Two other choices are important, however.
13. Click Checking Mail.
14. *Save Password*: If this is checked, the password will be saved in encrypted form in a file on your computer, so when you check for new mail you will not have to enter the password.
15. *Leave mail on server:* If this is checked, new mail will be downloaded but a copy will stay on the mail server computer. At some point the mail has to be deleted from there, so at least one of the programs you use to read mail has to have this unchecked.
16. When you are done, click OK.

B. SEND A MESSAGE

1. Start Eudora.
2. Click the Message menu, then New Message.
3. Type in your own email address.
4. Press the Tab key, or click with the mouse to the right of the word Subject.
5. Type `just testing.`
6. Press the Tab key until the blinking cursor is in the lower text area, or click the mouse once in that area.
7. Type `body of my message.`
8. Click the Send button, or the menu Message, Send Immediately.

C. ADD A NAME TO THE ADDRESSBOOK

1. Click the menu Tools, Addressbook, or the Addressbook icon (third from the right). (Eudora 2: Window, Nicknames menu)
2. In the lower left of the Addressbook window, click the New button.
3. Type your first name.
4. Click OK or press the Enter key.
5. Type your email address.
6. Repeat these steps with at least one friend's address. Click the New button to start.
7. Click the File, Save menu to save your change.

SEND AN EMAIL MESSAGE USING THE ADDRESSBOOK ALIAS

An alias is a name that stands for something else. You can now use your first name to send messages, rather than type your full email address.

1. Click the Message, New Message menu.
2. Type your first name in the To: line.
3. Press the Tab key once.
4. Type `message 2` in the Subject line.
5. Click the Send button.

USE THE ADDRESSBOOK ITSELF TO SEND A MESSAGE

1. Click the menu Tools, Addressbook, (Eudora 2: Window, Nicknames menu) or the Addressbook icon (third from the right).
2. Click your name (left side of window).
3. Click the To: button.
4. Tab to the Subject line and type `more junk`.
5. Click the Send button.

SEND A CARBON COPY (CC:) WITH A MESSAGE

1. Click the menu Tools, Addressbook, (Eudora 2: Window, Nicknames menu) or the Addressbook icon (third from the right).
2. Click the Message, New Message menu.
3. Type your friend's name in the To: line.
4. Press the Tab key once.
5. Type `testing carbon copy` in the Subject line.
6. Press the Tab key once.
7. Type your own first name in the Cc: line.
8. Click the Send button.

D. SEND AN ATTACHED FILE

1. Click the Message, New Message menu.
2. Type your first name in the To: line.
3. Click the Message, Attach File menu.
4. Look for any file with .txt at the end. Click that file name.
5. Click Open (Eudora 2: OK)
6. The attachments line of your message will now read something like c:\eudora\changes.txt
7. Click in the subject line and type `testing attachments`
8. Click the Send button.

CHECK FOR NEW MESSAGES

1. Click File, Check Mail.
2. The Eudora program will connect to the mail server computer and download any new mail. The inbox should open.
3. If the inbox is small, double-click its title bar (to the right of the word In) to expand it.)
4. For each message you see Who it came from, the Date it came, and the Subject, among other things.
5. Double-click the message titled just testing to open it.
6. You will see some header information, then the subject and the message ("body of my message")
7. Click Mailbox, In to see your messages again.

OPEN AN ATTACHMENT

1. In the Inbox, double-click the message with the subject testing attachments.
2. The attached file will appear in the message.
3. Double-click the icon for the file. (Eudora 2: Double-click the line which reads "Attachment converted...") This will start the program that created the file and load it into that program.
4. Click File, Exit to close this program.

DELETE A MESSAGE

1. While you are reading a message, you can delete it by: pressing the Delete key; clicking on the Trash icon; or clicking Message, Delete. This sends the message to a "trash" bin. You can still recover these messages, until you exit the program, when the trash is "emptied."
2. Click Message, Delete to get rid of this message.

REPLY TO A MESSAGE

1. Click the message which says "message 2"
2. Click the Message, Reply menu.
3. A new message comes up addressed to the person it came from (you). It quotes the original and has the subject Re: message 2
4. Type `reply to message 2` and press the Enter key a few times.
5. Click the Send button.

E. CREATE A MAILBOX

This creates a mailbox in your Eudora program where you can store messages. The "mailbox" is a file on your personal computer. It does not affect the mail computer where your incoming mail is stored.

1. Click the Mailbox, New menu.
2. Type `Saved Messages.`
3. Click OK or press the Enter key.

TRANSFER A MESSAGE TO YOUR NEW MAILBOX

1. Click message 2 in the inbox.
2. Click the Transfer menu, then click Saved Messages.
3. This message has been transferred to your new mailbox.

OPEN A DIFFERENT MAILBOX

1. Click Mailbox, then Saved Messages.
2. You will see the message you transferred there.

NETSCAPE (VERSION 3 OR 4)

The exercises are written for Netscape 3. Differences between versions 3 and 4 are noted under each section.

F. SET UP NETSCAPE

You must first have access to the Internet on your computer, and an email account. Before you get started ask your computer administrator to tell you the following: your login name, email address, pop server, smtp server, and news server. The instructions below cover only the essentials of getting Netscape to the point where it will send and receive mail. There are many settings not discussed below.

NETSCAPE 3

1. Click the Options, Mail and News Preferences menu item.
2. Click the Identity tab.
3. *Name*: Type your full name. *Email address*: Type your full email address, e.g. john.doe@university.edu or john.doe@mycompany.com
4. *Reply to address*: enter your email address.
5. Click the Servers tab.
6. *Outgoing Mail (SMTP) Server*: see above for Eudora.
7. *Incoming Mail (POP3) Server*: Type the name of the mail computer, something like `pop3.mycompany.com` or `computer.university.edu`
8. POP3 user name: Type your login name.
9. News (NNTP) server: This is the name of the computer that carries Usenet discussion groups, something like `news.mycompany.com` or `news.university.edu`
10. Click OK.

NETSCAPE 4

1. Start Netscape.
2. Click the Edit, Preferences menu.
3. Click the plus sign (+) by Mail and Groups.
4. Click Identity. Same as Netscape 3.
5. Click Messages. Uncheck the box next to By default, send HTML messages. Otherwise your mail will go out formatted as Web pages.
6. Click Mail Server.
7. *Mail server user name*: Type your login name.
8. *Outgoing and Incoming mail*: Same as Netscape 3.
9. Click Groups Server.
10. *Discussion Groups server*: This is the name of the computer that carries Usenet discussion groups, e.g. `news.mycompany.com` or `news.university.edu`
11. Click OK.

G. SEND A MESSAGE

1. Click File, New Mail Message. (Netscape 4: Communicator, Message Center, New Message
2. Type in your own email address.
3. Press the Tab key, or click with the mouse to the right of the word Subject.
4. Type `just testing`.
5. Press the Tab key until the blinking cursor is in the lower text area, or click the mouse once in that area.
6. Type `body of my message`.
7. Click the Send button, or the menu File, Send Now.

H. ADD A NAME TO THE ADDRESSBOOK

1. Click the menu Window, Addressbook, (Netscape 4: Communicator, Addressbook).
2. Click Item, Add User. (Netscape 4: File, New Card)
3. Type your nickname (first name), name, and email address. Use Tab key between each, and Enter key at the end. (Netscape 4: Type at least the first name and email address.)
4. Repeat these steps with at least one friend's address.
5. Click the File, Close menu.

SEND AN EMAIL MESSAGE USING THE ADDRESSBOOK ALIAS

An alias is a name that stands for something else. You can now use your first name to send messages, rather than type your full email address.

1. Click File, New Mail Message (Netscape 4: Communicator, Message Center, New Message)
2. Type your first name in the To: line.
3. Press the Tab key once.
4. Type `message 2` in the Subject line.
5. Click the Send button. Netscape will tell you that you haven't typed anything in the message. Click OK.

USE THE ADDRESSBOOK ITSELF TO SEND A MESSAGE

1. Click Window, Addressbook (Netscape 4: Communicator, Addressbook)
2. Right-click your name and select New Message.
3. Tab to the Subject line and type `more junk`.
4. Click the Send button.

SEND A CARBON COPY (CC:) WITH A MESSAGE

1. Start a message as the last exercise, but send it to your friend's address.
2. Press the Tab key once.
3. Type `testing carbon copy` in the Subject line.
4. Click in the Cc: line.
5. Type your own first name in the Cc: line.
6. Click the Send button.

SEND AN ATTACHED FILE

1. Start a message to yourself as above.
2. Click in the Subject line and type `testing attachments`.
3. Click the Attach button, then Attach File. (Netscape 4: Attach button, then File.)
4. Click the button next to the text box with Program to go up one level.
5. Click the readme.txt file then Open, then OK.
6. The attachments line of your message will now show readme.txt (In Netscape 4 this line may be hidden if the address line is showing.)
7. Click the Send button.

CHECK FOR NEW MESSAGES

1. Click Window, Netscape Mail. (Netscape 4: Communicator, Get Mail)
2. The Netscape program will connect to the mail server computer and download any new mail. The inbox should open.
3. For each message you see who sent it (Sender), the Date it came, and the Subject, among other things.
4. Double-click the message titled "just testing" to open it.
5. You will see some header information, then the subject and the message ("body of my message").
6. Click Mailbox, In to see your messages again.

OPEN AN ATTACHMENT

1. In the Inbox, double-click the message with the subject testing attachments.
2. The attached file will appear in the message. If you attached a file that was created with a program such as Word, you will see a link in the message to that file. When you double-click the link, that program will start and the file will be loaded.
3. Click File, Exit to close the program.

DELETE A MESSAGE

1. While you are reading a message, you can delete it by: pressing the Delete key or by clicking the onscreen Delete button.

REPLY TO A MESSAGE

1. Click the message which says "message 2"
2. Click the Message, Reply menu. (Netscape 4: Message, Reply to Sender.
3. A new message comes up addressed to the person it came from (you). It quotes the original and has the subject Re: message 2
4. Type `reply to message 2`
5. Click the Send button.

I. CREATE A MAILBOX

This creates a mailbox in your Netscape program where you can store messages. The "mailbox" is a file on your personal computer. It does not affect the mail computer where your incoming mail is stored.

1. Click the File, New folder menu. (Netscape 4:
2. Type `Saved Messages.`
3. Click OK or press the Enter key.

TRANSFER A MESSAGE TO YOUR NEW MAILBOX

1. Click once on message 2 in the inbox.
2. Click the Message menu, then Move. (Netscape 4: Message, File).
3. Click the Saved Messages folder. This message has been transferred to your new mailbox.

OPEN A DIFFERENT MAILBOX

1. Click Saved Messages folder. (Netscape 4: Communicator, Message Center, Saved Messages.)
2. You will see the message you transferred there.

II. Problem-Solving

- Create a signature file, then test it.
- Create a filter so that all mail with your address in the header drops into a specific mailbox. Then test it by sending yourself a message.

III. Thought and Discussion

- Brainstorm with your class to come up with five ways that email can be used in a clinical setting.
- Do people become more emotional when using email?
- What precautions can you take to prevent email with clinical information from being read by an unauthorized person?

Readings From the Net

(Links available at http://NewWindPub.com/workbook)

Email Programs

A Beginner's Guide to Effective Email	http://www.webfoot.com/advice/email.top.html	Style guide showing you the fine points of email.
Eudora e-mail program	http://www.netspot.unisa.edu.au/eudora/contents.html	How to set it up, what to do with rejected messages, etc. Images showing what Eudora looks like.
Unix Pine email program	http://www.snre.umich.edu/pinedocs/pine.internet.intro.html	Also shows you what the screen looks like. Short and to the point.

Chapter 6: Bookmarks: Beam Me Back, Scotty!

How confidently I had overlooked all this: rocks, bugs, rain. What else was I missing?
Annie Dillard, An American Childhood

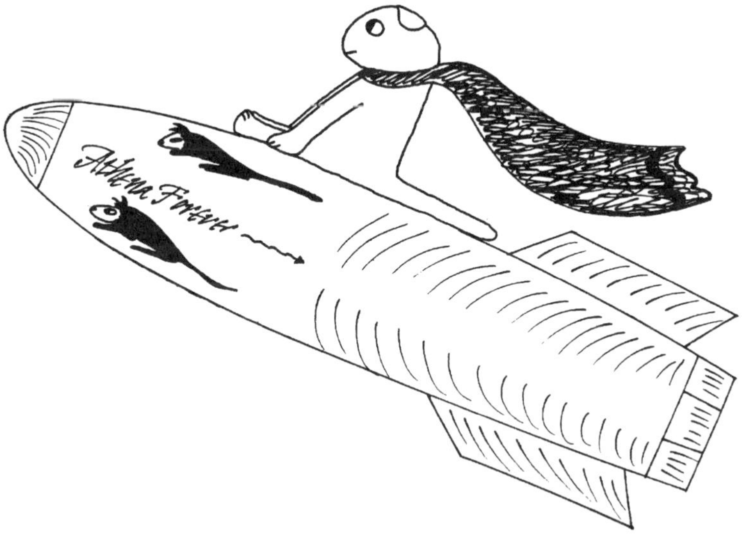

IN THIS CHAPTER

- bookmarks
- drag and drop
- folders
- import
- nesting
- properties
- separators

Most of us come out of school with the impression that being smart means knowing things. Knowledge of basic information is important, but so is knowing where to look up something that you haven't memorized.

On the Internet it is often easy to find a site; but how do you get back there a week or a year later, when all you remember is that it had something to do with pediatrics? The Web has approximately one hundred million sites, and they continue to appear at an exponential rate. How do you keep track of those which are critical to your specialty or area of interest?

Bookmarks

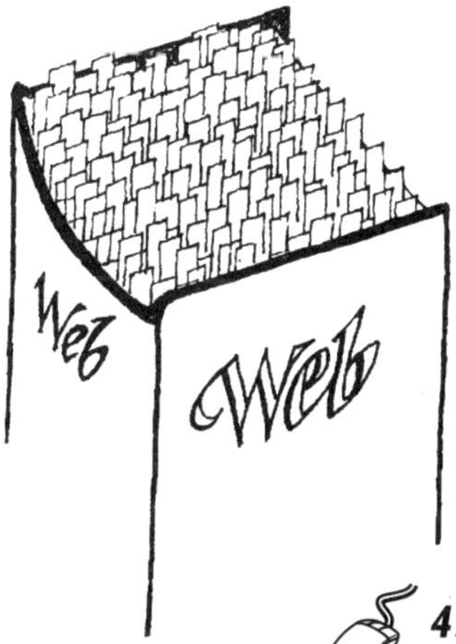

Most Web browsers allow you to save a pointer to a Web site, called a bookmark. (In Explorer they are called *Favorites*; in AOL, *Favorite Places*; in Compuserve, *Hotlists*. But they all function similarly.) When you want to return to a site, you simply click the bookmark for that site, and the browser will take you there. You don't have to type the address; in fact, you don't even have to know what the address is.

Think of the Web as a gigantic book, with millions of pages. When you see a chapter or page that you want to look at again, you put a marker, a bookmark, there. To return, you open the book at that marker.

Not surprisingly, the bookmark function in Netscape has changed significantly with each version of the program. But in Netscape 3 and 4 basic functions remain the same; once you understand these, you will be able to work much more efficiently on the Web.

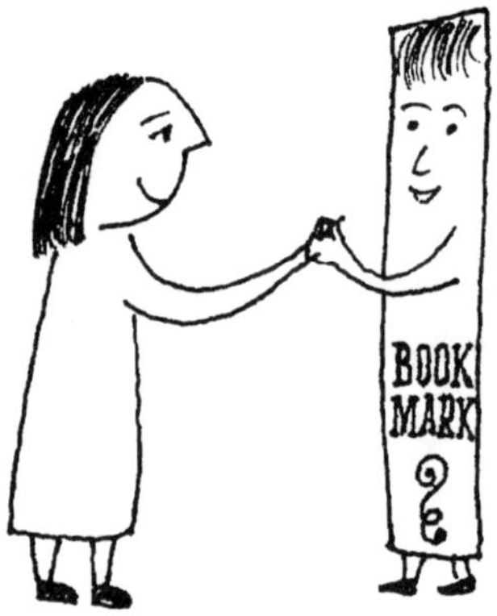

Creating Bookmarks

To create a bookmark, click the Bookmark menu item, then Add Bookmark. (In Netscape 4, you can "file" a bookmark to a specific folder.) Nothing seems to happen, but Netscape has put the name and address of the current Web page at the bottom of the list. When you click the Bookmark menu again, you will see it there.

Visiting Bookmarks

Visiting a bookmark is simple: click the Bookmark menu, then the name of the site you want to visit. Netscape will automatically take you there. Remember that Internet addresses change, however, so an address that worked last month may not work today. (About forty addresses out of three hundred in my *Pocket Guide to the Medical Internet* changed after only six months.) Some sites will automatically forward you to the new page, and others put up a notice of the new address. But in some cases you will be left floating in the ether.

Arranging Bookmarks

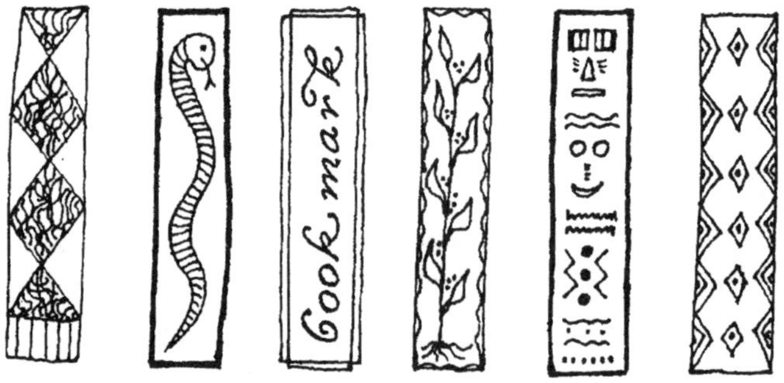

Many people never get past the stage of simply saving bookmarks to a list. They end up with a list of fifty or a hundred sites, and every time they want to visit one they have to look through the entire list to find it. But that's unnecessary: Netscape gives you a couple of very useful tools for working with your bookmarks.

Folders

Netscape allows you to put similar bookmarks into folders. A folder is like a directory on the computer. You can name your folders (e.g. Pediatrics, or Entertainment, or Stores). Once you create a folder you can then put bookmarks there, either by "filing" them with Netscape 4 or by dragging and dropping them into the folder.

Viewing Bookmarks Within Folders

To see a folder and its bookmarks, you click the Bookmarks menu. You will see a list of folders (these will have a triangle to the right of the folder name) or single bookmarks.

Moving Several Bookmarks

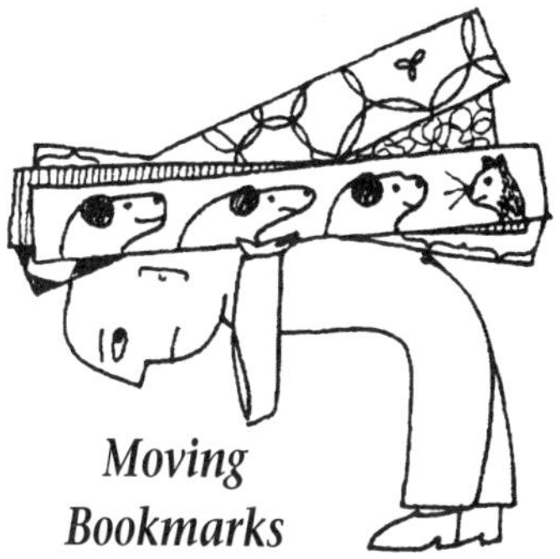

Moving Bookmarks

In many Windows programs, holding down the Ctrl (Control) key allows you to select more than one item. (For example, in the Eudora email program you can select more than one address from the nickname list.) Similarly, holding down the Shift key allows you to select everything between two items. After you create bookmarks and folders, try moving them around. Using the Shift key or the Control key, select several at once and then drag and drop them into a folder.

Cut and Paste a Bookmark

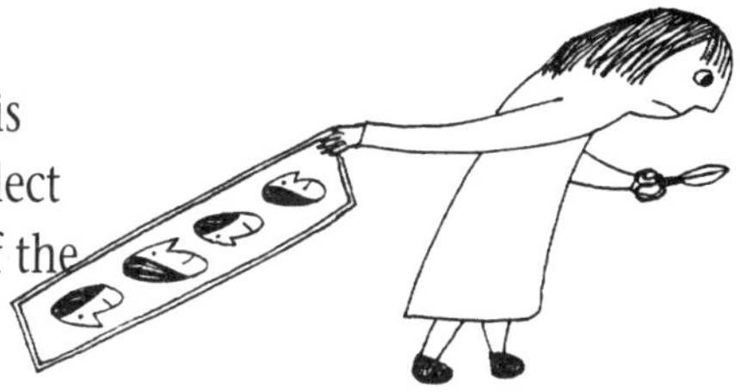

Another way to move and arrange bookmarks is by cutting and pasting. This becomes especially easy with the mouse. You right-click a bookmark and select Cut, then right-click where you want it to go and select Paste. This is one of the most useful functions in Windows 95.

Move and Nest Folders

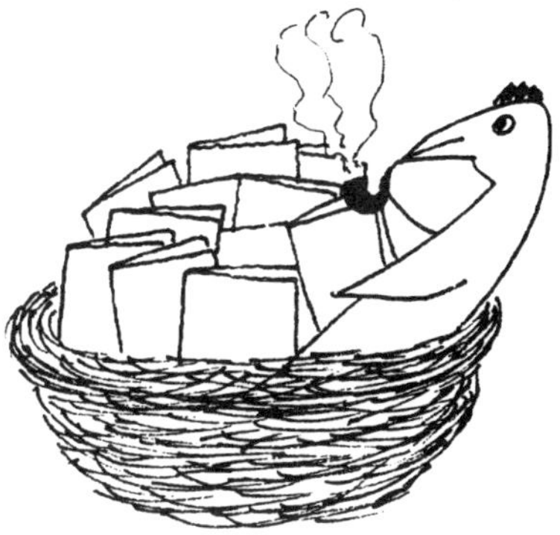

You can move a folder with the same techniques described above, and put it inside another folder as you would put a box inside another box. This is called nesting. And imagine the possibilities of organization it gives you. Instead of having a list of two hundred bookmarks to scroll through each time you want to find one, you place those two hundred into ten groups of twenty each.

The Watchmaker's Principle

Organizing work, ideas, or information into categories is a useful technique in general, quite apart from computers. Suppose that to build a watch takes one hundred individual steps. You can start from step one and go to the end, but if you make a mistake you have to start over.

The other way is to group the steps into ten categories of ten steps each. For example, building the hands takes ten steps. When an accident occurs, you never lose more than ten steps. It also makes it easier to think about the process.

For example, health care has devised several ways to group the process of thinking or charting about patients. A SOAP note is a good example. Rather than try to put the entire process of thinking about the patient into one long list, you categorize your thoughts and notes into subjective, objective, assessment, and plan.

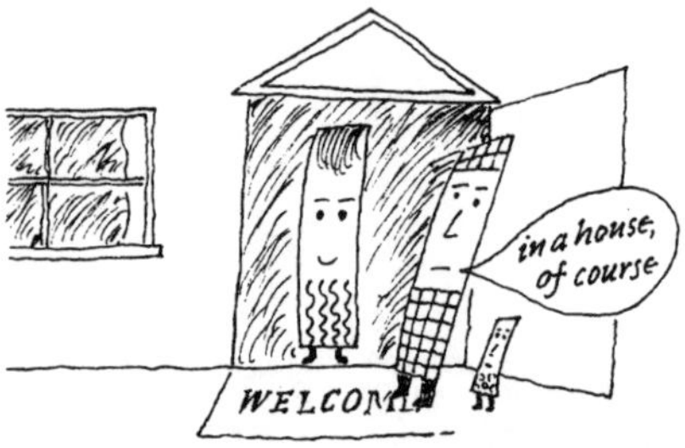

Where Do Bookmarks Live?

The bookmark list is actually an HTML (Web) document, titled bookmark.htm, that has taken up residence in the Netscape directory. You can open it from within the Netscape program, just as you would any other HTML file. You can also save the entire list to another directory, then edit it if necessary, and send it as an email attachment to a friend or colleague. This lets you share the research you have done in collecting resources.

Import

To bring information into one document from another.

Importing a Bookmark List

You can also import another person's bookmark list into your own, so you can take advantage of research and browsing that others have done.

Creating an Instant Web Page

Because your bookmark list is also an html file, you can use it to create a list of resources to go on the Web. This is the most painless way I know of to create a Web page with a list of links to Web sites.

Change the Name of a Bookmark

When you create a bookmark it will have the same name as the title of the Web page. But some Web pages don't have titles; for these you will see the address of the page, which doesn't help you very much when you are looking through the list. You can edit a bookmark name later to something that makes more sense to you.

Place A Bookmark on the Desktop

With Windows 95, you can drag a bookmark to the desktop, where it will become a shortcut. Then, you can double-click the shortcut to start your browser and go to that site. (Note that if you are using a home computer, you must first connect to your service provider before the browser will be able to download the Web page.)

No matter how well other methods become for finding sites on the Web, you will always want to mark your own spots. "Every original mind, in whatever field she works, is an explorer." (Ashley Montague, *Growing Young*)

EXERCISES

Each lettered exercise is independent.
(Links available at http://NewWindPub.com/workbook)

I. Guided Practice

A. SAVE A BOOKMARK

1. Start Netscape or Explorer.
2. Go to a different page than the home page.
3. Click Bookmarks, Add Bookmark (Explorer: Favorites, Add to Favorites.)
4. Go to the Home page.
5. Try your bookmark by clicking Bookmarks, then the name of the new bookmark.

CREATE A FOLDER

1. Click Bookmarks, Go to Bookmarks (Netscape 4: Bookmarks, Edit Bookmarks; Explorer: Favorites, Organize Favorites.)
2. Click Item, Insert Folder. (Explorer: Right-click. Select New, Folder.)
3. Type `Medical Directories`
4. Click OK (Explorer: Close)

FILE A BOOKMARK (NETSCAPE 4 AND EXPLORER)

1. Create a folder named Medical Search
2. Go to http://pride-sun.poly.edu
3. Click Bookmarks, File Bookmark. (Explorer: Favorites, Create In.)
4. Move the mouse pointer over the Medical Search folder, and click.

DRAG A BOOKMARK INTO A FOLDER

1. Go to http://www.medmatrix.org
2. Add a bookmark to this page.
3. Click Bookmarks, Go to Bookmarks. (Netscape 4: Bookmarks, Edit Bookmarks; Explorer: Favorites, Organizc Favorites.)
4. Drag the bookmark for the Medical Matrix and drop it on your Medical Directories folder.
5. Click File, Close. (Explorer: Close)
6. Click the Home button to return there.
7. Click Bookmarks, Medical Directories, Medical Matrix to test.

PUT A FOLDER WITHIN A FOLDER

1. Create a folder named Medical Specialties.
2. Create a folder named AIDS.
3. Go to http://www.teleport.com/~celinec/aids.shtml
4. Create a bookmark for this page.
5. Click Bookmarks, Go to Bookmarks (Netscape 4: Bookmarks, Edit Bookmarks); Explorer: Favorites, Organize Favorites.)
6. Drag the bookmark titled AIDS Resource List into the AIDS folder.
7. Drag the AIDS folder into the Medical Specialties folder.
8. Click File, Close.
9. Click the Home button to return there.
10. Test your folders: Click Bookmarks, Medical Specialties, AIDS, AIDS Resource List.

CHANGE A BOOKMARK NAME

1. Click Bookmarks, Go to... (Netscape 4: Bookmarks, Edit; Explorer: Favorites, Organize Favorites.)
2. Click the Medical Directories Folder.
3. Right-click Medical Matrix.
4. Click Properties.
5. Type `Matrix.`
6. Click OK.

B. RIGHT-CLICK TO CREATE A BOOKMARK

1. Go to http://www.HealthAtoZ.com
2. Right-click anywhere on the Web page.
3. Click Add Bookmark.(Explorer: Add to Favorites.)
4. Click Bookmarks to see the change.

C. RIGHT-CLICK TO CREATE A SHORTCUT (WINDOWS 95 ONLY)

1. Go to http://www.achoo.com
2. Right-click anywhere on the Web page.
3. Click Internet Shortcut. (Netscape 4: Create Shortcut)
4. Click OK.
5. Right-click an empty part of the taskbar at the bottom of the screen.
6. Click Minimize all Windows.
7. Double-click one of the new shortcuts.

II. Problem-Solving

- Save your bookmarks to a file, then send it to another person to see if she can import them into her list.
- Mail your bookmark file to yourself and then open it as a Web page.

III. Thought and Discussion

- How can you store bookmarks so they will be available no matter where you are working?
- How might you set up bookmarks so other people can share them?

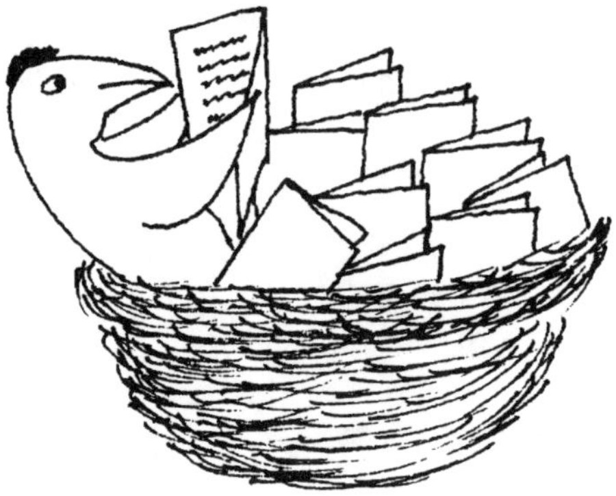

Readings from the Net

(Links available from http://NewWindPub.com/wkbook)

Bookmarks

Bookmarks	http://www.cnet.com/Resources/Tech/Advisers/Bookmark	Discussion and how-to.

Part Two:
Medical Information

Directories

Searching

MEDLINE and CINAHL

Patient Education

Medical Journals and News

Medical Sites

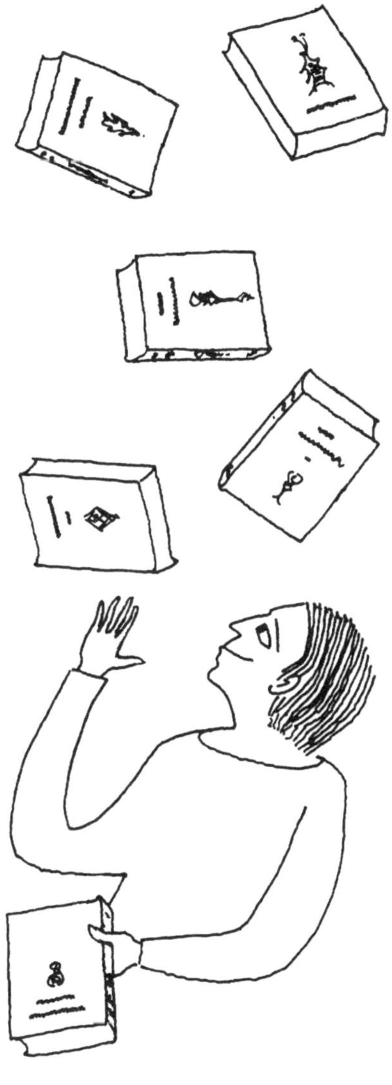

After finishing Part Two, you will be able to:

- *Use a subject directory to find medical sites*
- *Use search engines to find medical sites*
- *Search MEDLINE and CINAHL for article citations*
- *Find patient education materials on the Internet*
- *Find medical journals on the Internet*
- *Find sites in your specialty*

Chapter 7: Directories

I do not know what I may appear to the world, but to myself I seem to have been only like a boy playing on the sea-shore, and diverting myself now and then finding a smoother pebble or a prettier shell than ordinary while all the great ocean of truth lay all undiscovered before me.

Sir Isaac Newton

IN THIS CHAPTER

annotations
citing an Internet source
directory
layout
MeSH
metadirectory
peer review
ratings
specialty
sublevels

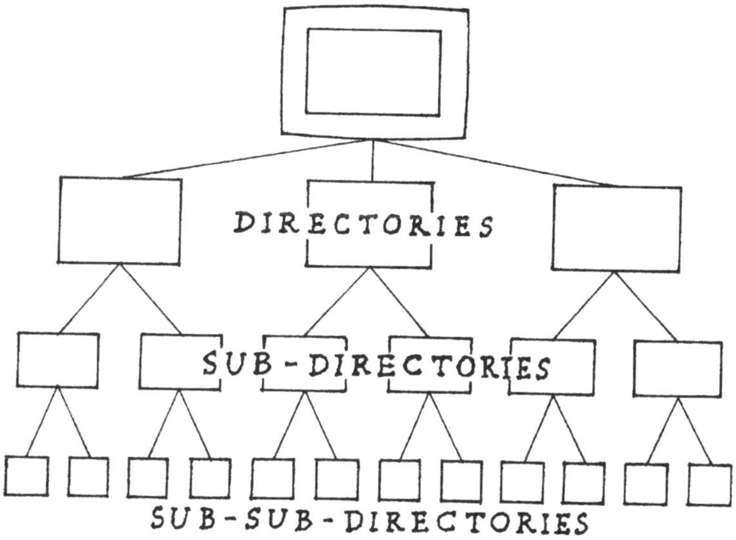

The Internet is bewildering partly because of its sheer size. If we can't get through a few magazines every month, how am we going to ever manage among millions of Web sites? The open secret is that it's not necessary to be conversant with a million, or even a dozen sites. One good directory is sufficient.

A directory (also called subject index, guide, or tree) is a list of sites. The Yellow Pages telephone directory, for example, is a list of businesses. Look in the Yellow Pages under Computer, and you see further categories: Computer Dealers, Computer Graphics, Computer Training. Each of these areas will have its own list.

On the Internet, some directories list Web sites on all topics, and others are limited to special topics, such as health care. General directories will often have a section covering health care, so don't overlook them as a good source of information.

Directories and Search Engines

Most online directories are searchable, meaning that you can look for an entry by typing a word into a box and making a computer look for the word, rather than having to browse through page after page of lists. Because searching is an important topic and search skills are critical to using the Internet effectively, the next chapter is devoted entirely to search engines. But keep in mind that the distinction is fuzzy: most directories include some kind of search engine.

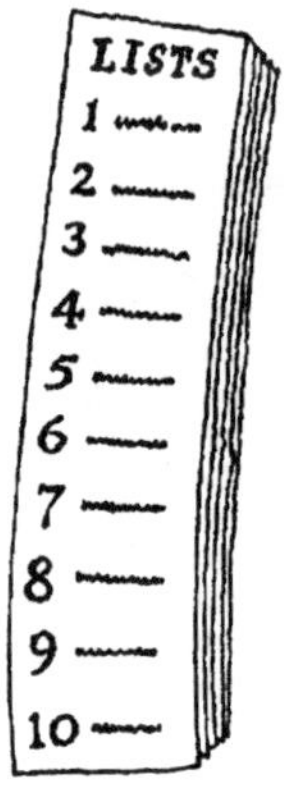

Lists of Lists

You can also find directories of directories. Because these are one level removed from the actual information you are looking for, they are called metadirectories. The best metadirectory related to medicine is the Hardin MetaDirectory of Internet Health Sources, from the Hardin Library of Health Sciences at the University of Iowa (http://www.arcade.uiowa.edu/hardin-www/md.html) which gives medical directories arranged by specialty (Anesthesiology, Dentistry, Pediatrics, etc.). Hardin categorizes them into three types: short, medium, or long, depending on how many sites each one contains. To do an in-depth search on a subject, pick a long directory; for a quick introduction, pick a short one.

Choosing A Directory

Medical directories are very different from each other. Their criteria, organization, screen presentation, search capacity, number of entries, review board, annotations, method and frequency of updating, and availability all vary from one to the next. The best strategy for working efficiently on the Internet is to browse a wide range of directories, then choose one that suits your needs best and spend some time becoming familiar with it.

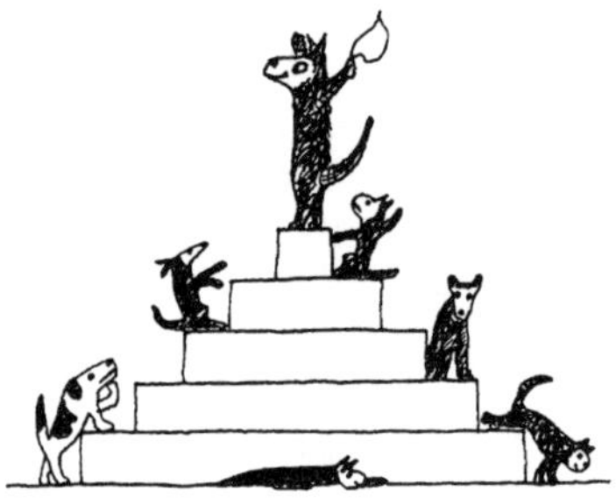

Number of Levels

By "levels" I mean the number of pages you have to click through before you get to links to other sites. Some directories have only two levels: the table of contents, and the actual list. MedMark (http://medmark.bit.co.kr) is a good example. Each specialty link (Endocrinology, Nephrology) takes you to a long list of sites. To see a directory that uses multiple levels, take a look at Achoo (http://www.achoo.com).

Notice that there is a trade-off in the time it takes to find a resource using each kind of directory. MedMark takes you to a list of sites right away, but you have to scroll down the page and actively read the entries to find a specific resource. With Achoo you have to click through multiple pages, but once there, you see sites related to a very specific topic.

Notes

Annotation
A short note or review.

Which is more useful in the Yellow Pages, the name and phone number for a business, or a full-page advertisement that tells the hours it is open, what services it offers, and how to get there? Advertisements can be useful because they contain extra information. We read reviews of movies and books for the same reason, to get more information than a simple title provides.

In a directory these are usually called reviews. Reviews are very useful for online directories and books about the Net. Most of us are too busy to personally visit a hundred sites to find a single one, especially when using a modem. In my first book (*An Internet Guide for the Health Professional*) each entry for a site had a short review so that readers could get a quick impression of the contents.

Not all directories have reviews. MedMark is an example of a list without them. Although the list is extensive, you have to visit each site to find out just what is there.

To see a medical directory with reviews, go to the Medical Matrix (http://www.medmatrix.org). You will find a succinct description of the contents of each site. I recommend the Medical Matrix as an excellent starting point for searching the medical Internet.

Peer Review...

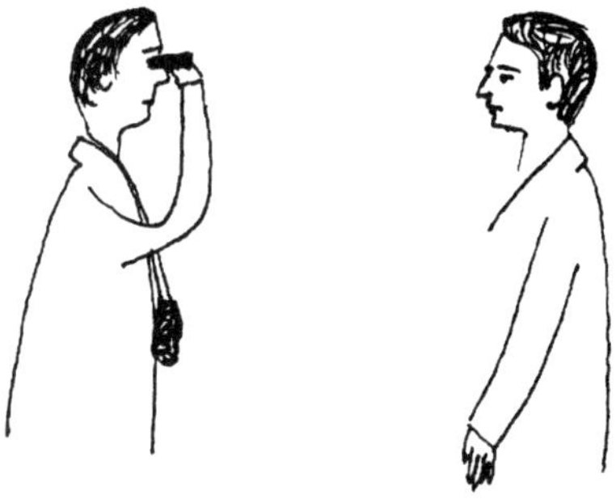

The Medical Matrix also uses peer review, which adds to the authority of their recommendations. This means that each site has been reviewed by someone in the medical field (a peer), who has decided that the contents of the site are authoritative. Peer review has long been used by reputable journals to ensure that articles which are published meet the highest standards.

...versus Self-Publishing

The alternative to peer review is self-publishing; much of the best and the worst you see on the Internet falls into this category. When a person puts a Web site up without anyone else being involved, he avoids editorial interference. Nobody can revise or censor or change what he wants to say. Of course, nobody can correct factual mistakes or improve the writing either.

Self-publishing didn't originate with the Internet. But because the costs of publishing on the Web are small to non-existent, more and more people are putting up material of questionable value. You can still rely on the name of established journals, for example the *New England Journal of Medicine*, to ensure factual accuracy. But check your sources; many sites may have high-sounding names and little else to guarantee their authority. Use your professional judgment.

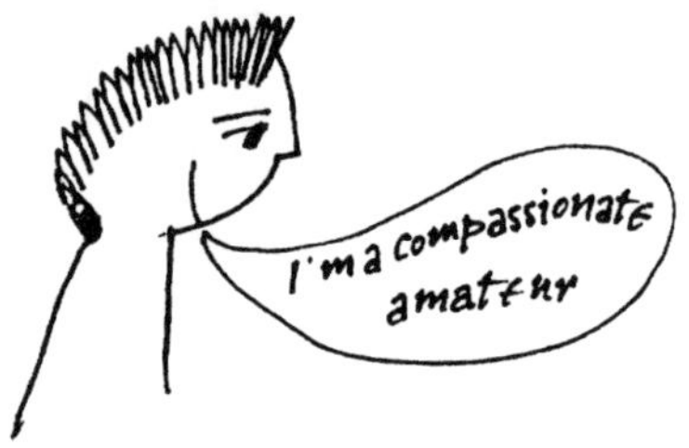

Compassionate Amateurs

Anyone who has been a patient knows that it is often difficult to find materials that are written for the non-professional. Not surprisingly, some of the most useful teaching materials on medical conditions have been written by other patients. The experience of disease itself often generates a deep compassion for others in the same situation.

Although directories such as Matrix or MedWeb are a good place to start, you will often find excellent lists put together by non-professionals. These often contain more complete reviews of each site, well-organized lists of support organizations, and non-traditional approaches to medicine. The best example of a directory that was started by non-professionals is Med Help International (http://medhlp.netusa.net), a superb Web site with a medical advisory board for peer review, extensive resources for patients, a Web library, forums, chat, and a 6,000-word medical dictionary.

Different Ways of Classifying Medical Information

Even in a professional field such as medicine, there are different ways to organize information. Most medical directories classify by medical specialty: anesthesiology, cardiology, dermatology, etc. The Medical Matrix and Hardin follow this traditional scheme closely.

> **MeSH**
>
> Medical Subject Headings, from the Library of Medicine.

Several directories use the National Library of Medicine's MeSH (Medical Subject Headings; see Chapter 9) to arrange their sites. CliniWeb (http://www.ohsu.edu/cliniweb) allows you to browse through the MeSH hierarchy, starting with the top two categories, anatomy and diseases. Karolinska Institute (http://www.mic.ki.se/Diseases) also organizes by MeSH.

Alphabetical

Not all arrangements are what they seem. On the Karolinska Institute's page is a button for an "Alphabetical List of Diseases." But clicking on "achondroplasia," for example, leads to a page which lists all sites related to musculoskeletal disorders. Then you will have to look through that page to find achondroplasia. In other words, the alphabetical list doesn't lead you to sites related to that disease, rather to a page which covers a wider variety of topics.

True alphabetical lists of medical sites are not very common. Exceptions are dictionaries or glossaries, such as Dr. Schueler's On-line Medical Glossary (http://www.drschueler.com/glossary/glossary.htm) or the subsections of the Collaborative Hypertext of Radiology (http://chorus.rad.mcw.edu/chorus.html). Patient education sites such as Health Explorer (http://www.healthexplorer.com) often have alphabetical lists of diseases.

Type of Document

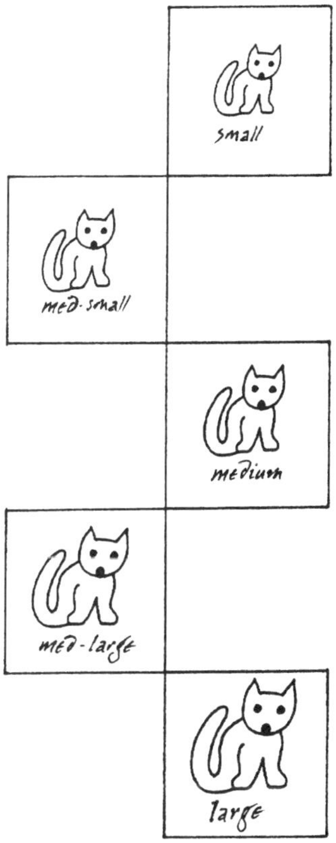

A natural way to organize a collection of materials is by type of document: newspaper report, journal article, book, videotape, mailing list, newsgroup, and so on. If you want to find news in the public library, for example, you go to the newspaper rack. Medical sites will often have a category for news, and smaller directories devoted to an individual specialty have pages showing mailing lists, newsgroups, and books about the specialty.

This kind of classification has limits. The keyword area of MedWeb (http://www.gen.emory.edu/MEDWEB/keyword.html) shows several types of document: bibliographies, calendars, databases, electronic publications, indices (directories). It further classifies material into brochures, catalogs, documents, guidelines, lists, software, tutorials. Take these classifications with a grain of salt. A single document could be a tutorial, a white paper, an electronic document, an electronic publication, a document, a handout, a report, a manuscript, or a textbook, depending on who did the classifying.

Audience

Yet another way to organize is by the type of audience a document was written for. The home page of the Virtual Hospital (http://vh.radiology.uiowa.edu) has links to two sections, one for healthcare providers and the other for patients, with the material arranged accordingly.

In practice there are few directories which use one system of classification exclusively. In the Matrix, for example, the top level includes Specialties, Marketplace, Literature, and Education. In HealthAtoZ (http://www.HealthAtoZ.com) are categories such as Medicine, Men's Health, Consulting, and Alternative Medicine. Version 3 of Achoo (http://www.achoo.com) has Human Health, Business of Health, and Organizations as the top three categories.

Citing an Internet Source

Increasingly, Internet sources will be cited in bibliographies. The following examples are based on *Electronic Styles*, by Li and Crane. (http://www.uvm.edu/~ncrane/estyles).

> **Citation**
>
> A reference in a library card catalog to a book or article.

Here is an example of the American Psychological Association (APA) Embellished Style:

> Pritzker, T. J. (No date). An Early fragment from central Nepal [Online]. Available: http://www.ingress.com/~astanart/pritzker/pritzker.html [1995, June 8].

And here is an example of the Modern Language Association (MLA) Embellished Style:

> Pritzker, Thomas J. An Early Fragment from Central Nepal. N.D. Online. Ingress Communications. Available: http://www.ingress.com/~astanart/pritzker/pritzker.html. 8 June 1995.

When you cite documents on the Web, think about the lifetime of the publication. Web addresses are not static. If a large number of citations are Web pages, the addresses may change in a few years, leaving the references unavailable to readers.

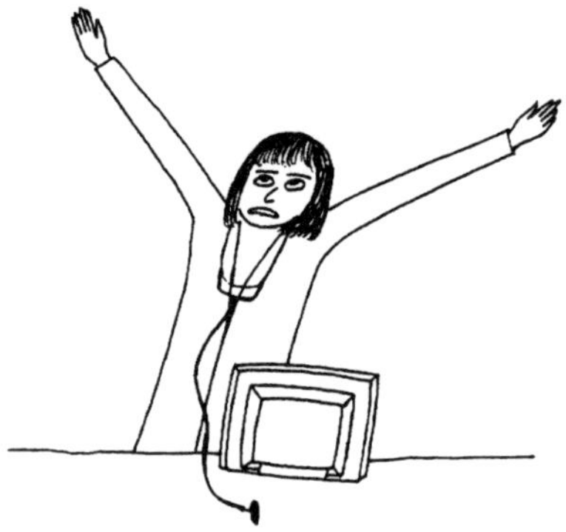

Digital despair

Computerized Searching

Though computer programs are being developed to scan and analyze text, we are not quite to the stage where a computer can intelligently read a document and decide exactly what the subject is, what categories it ought to go under, and what topics are related to it. The advantage of a directory is the work that an intelligent human being put into organizing and annotating the resources.

Although no comprehensive, standard method exists for classifying and searching for medical information, there is an alternative to endless browsing through subject directories. In the next chapter we see that with a search engine you can simply type in a word or phrase and the engine will find sites that match. Subject guides are a traditional way of looking for something, whereas search engines use the power of computerized databases to rapidly sift through vast quantities of data.

Subject Directories (Medical)

(Links available at http://NewWindPub.com/workbook)

Achoo	http://www.achoo.com	Over 7,500 sites. Hierarchy several levels deep, slow to navigate. Business & products as well as clinical sites; short reviews; good for searches on general terms.
CliniWeb	http://www.ohsu.edu/cliniweb	Uses MeSH hierarchy. No annotations. Links show sponsor for each site.
Cyberspace Medical Hospital	http://ch.nus.sg/CH/ch.html	From Singapore. Uses a hospital metaphor for organization. Can be slow.
Hardin Metadirectory	http://www.arcade.uiowa.edu/hardin-www/ md.html	Not searchable. 10-20 subject guides for each specialty, each list divided into large, medium and small guides. Good for a detailed search.
Harvard	http://www.med.harvard.edu/countway	Limited listings; easy to use. Go to Web resources. From Harvard's medical library.
HealthAtoZ	http://www.HealthAtoZ.com	Over 10,000 sites. Short reviews. Search on reviewed sites or entire database; search sub-categories. Advanced search; good for technical searches on single words.
HealthWeb	http://hsinfo.ghsl.nwu.edu:80/healthweb	Joint project among libraries. Short reviews.
Johns Hopkins	http://www.welch.jhu.edu/internet	Easy to navigate, but limited listings.
Kansas Univ. Medical Hospital	http://www.kumc.edu/service/dykes/ RRPAGES/rrintro.html	Directory; two-level. Very useful, long reviews, but not many sites listed.
Karolinska	http://www.mic.ki.se/Diseases/index.html	MeSH-categorized list of Web pages.
Martindale's Health	http://www-sci.lib.uci.edu/HSG/HSGuide.html	Awkward format. Large number of listings.
The Medical Matrix	http://www.medmatrix.org	Over 3,000 sites. Reviews and ratings by physician board. Simple structure. Poor search function.
MedExplorer	http://www.medexplorer.com	Compact format, one-line reviews.
MedMark	http://medmark.bit.co.kr	Lists by specialty. Large number of sites.
Medsite Navigator	http://www.medsitenavigator.com	Small but well-done, oriented to physicians.
MedWeb	http://www.cc.emory.edu/WHSCL/medweb.html	Over 8,000 sites. Keyword vs. alphabetical listing. Search looks at title, description.
MedGuide	http://www.medguide.net	Searchable directory; reviews; small number of listings in some categories.

Multi-Media Medical Library	http://www.med-library.com	Slow because of too many advertisements. Small to moderate number of sites listed.
North Memorial	http://www.nmmc.com/libweb/medstaff/mlinks.htm	Short but very well annotated list of links for each specialty.
Virtual Hospital	http://vh.radiology.uiowa.edu	Directory; info for prof. or public; primary clinical information; multimedia.
Virtual Library	http://golgi.harvard.edu/biopages/all.html	Directory; biosciences; long list; indentations for sub-categories.
WWW Virtual Library	http://golgi.harvard.edu/biopages/all.html	Alphabetical list of pages in the biomedical field; very large (226K) document.

Subject Directories(General)

Galaxy	http://galaxy.einet.net	Includes advanced searching. Very detailed hierarchy of topics.
Infoseek	http://www.infoseek.com	Advanced search functions.
PointCom	http://www.pointcom.com	Top 5% sites list. Can sort alphabetically, by date reviewed, content, or presentation.
Yahoo	http://www.yahoo.com	Most popular directory. Multiple sub-levels. You can create a personalized directory that shows a custom list of topics.

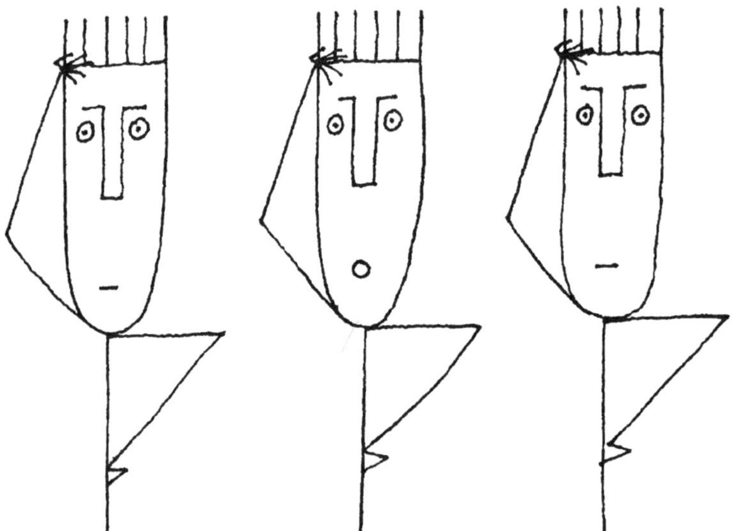

EXERCISES

Each lettered exercise is independent.
(Links available at http://NewWindPub.com/workbook)

I. Guided Practice

A. VISIT THE MEDICAL MATRIX

Visit a general medical directory and browse to find a full-text article.

1. Go to http://www.medmatrix.org
2. (Add a bookmark).
3. Scroll down and click Obstetrics.
4. Scroll down to read reviews.
5. Click practice Guidelines at CMA.
6. Choose an article and click full text.

B. VISIT MEDMARK

Vist a directory from Korea that uses frames.

1. Go to http://medmark.bit.co.kr
2. (Add a bookmark).
3. Click Hematology The file will take a minute, because it is large.
4. Click the various entries in the table of contents along the right side of the page.
5. For a review of aplastic anemia, click Diseases/ Conditions, then Aplastic anemia, introduction...

C. VISIT MEDWEB

This is a directory from Emory University which has been evolving continually, and which has a large number of sites listed.

1. Go to http://www.gen.emory.edu/MEDWEB
2. (Add a bookmark).
3. Click Keyword index.
4. Scroll down, click Geriatrics (By subcategory).
5. Note the organization of the page. Click Alzheimer's Disease.
6. Click the link titled Alzheimer's Web. (http://werple.mira.net.au/~dhs/ad.html).
7. Note the intermediate page that you see before you get to the Alzheimer Web page.
8. Click Enter Alzheimer Web! to see a topical arrangement of information about the disease.

D. VISIT THE HEALTH SECTION OF A GENERAL DIRECTORY

Some general directories have useful health or medical sections as well.

1. Go to http://www.excite.com
2. (Add a bookmark).
3. Click Health and Science
4. Note the organization of the page, which is more like a magazine than the previous directories.
5. Click a news story in the first section "Health and Science News" to see summaries from different newspapers, then click a headline to read an article.
6. Click the Back button to return to the Health and Science page.
7. Click Mental Health.
8. Scroll down the page. Note the ratings, the reviews, and the unreviewed sites.
9. Click editor's review for any site. This takes you to a page with all the reviews, and the site you chose at the top.

E. VISIT A SPECIALTY DIRECTORY (NURSING)

This is a directory of sites related to nursing. Similar directories exist for most specialties (though some are small). Look at chapter 12 for a site related to your specialty.

1. Go to http://www.lib.umich.edu/hw/nursing.html
2. (Add a bookmark)
3. Note the efficient hypertext paragraph below the graphic banner, linking to the medical library and school of nursing.
4. Click Organizations. Note the informative reviews of each site: a very useful aspect of directories.

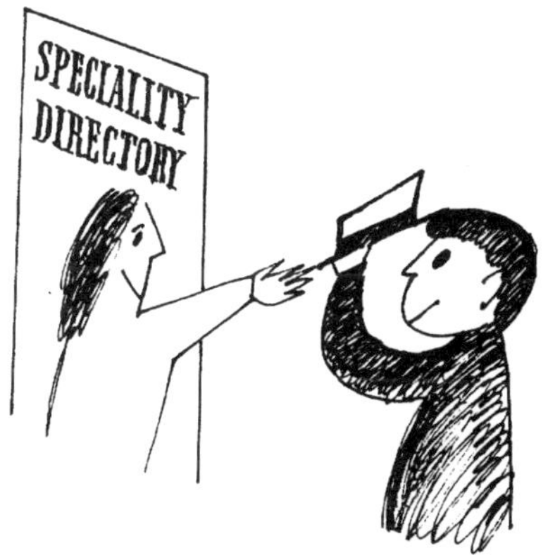

Problem-Solving

- Browse through the HealthAtoZ Web site (http://www.healthatoz.com) to see if you can find the listing for the Crohn's and Colitis Foundation of America (http://www.ccfa.org).
- Go to the Hardin Metadirectory (http://www.arcade.uiowa.edu/hardin-www/md.html) and compare several subject guides to geriatrics.

Thought and Discussion

- Write down a simple subject tree for your area of study or field (for example nursing or orthopedics) as if you were going to build a directory. Compare it to an online directory. Which makes more sense to you?
- Compare the Infoseek health list (http://www.infoseek.com/Health) with the Medical Matrix list (http://www.medmatrix.org). What are the strengths of each system of classification?
- Look at the table of contents for the policies in your institution. Describe the system of classification used. Is it by department, by type of procedure, by unit?

Chapter 8: Searching

Where observation is concerned, chance favours only the prepared mind.

Louis Pasteur

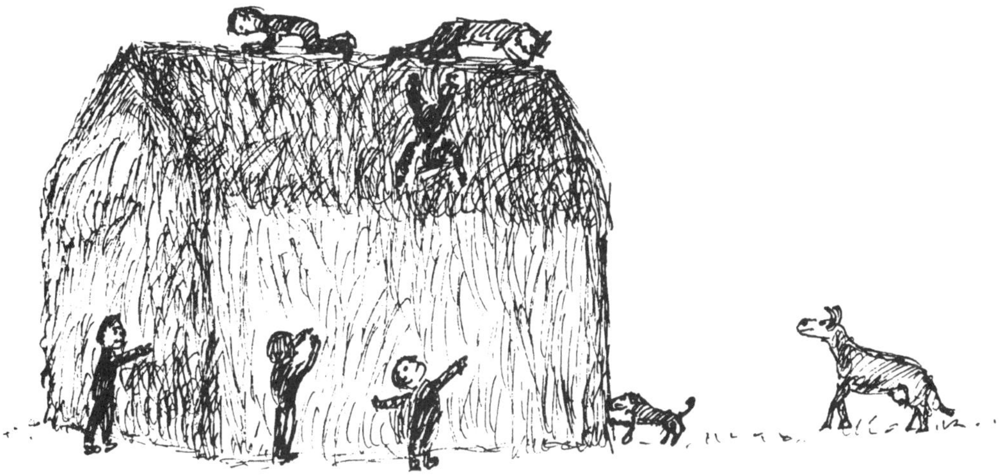

IN THIS CHAPTER

Boolean connectors
case sensitivity
full-text search
indexing
keyword search
metasearch
phrase search
proximity search
ranking
search engines
spiders, crawlers, bots, worms
title search
truncation

Search engines are Internet sites where you simply type in a word to find Web sites related to that word; this kind of magic has turned geeks and wonks into the idols of our time.

As with a directory, a search engine can be general, or limited to a topic. No special skills are needed to use a search engine; once there, click into a text box, type in the word(s), and click a Search button or press the Enter key. It's that easy. But understanding a few things about how searching is done will enable you to find better information in less time.

One of the largest and fastest general search engines is AltaVista (http://www.altavista.digital.com). Go there right now and give it a try. AltaVista is a database of some 30 million Web sites and millions of Usenet articles, yet it can run a search in a matter of a second or two. Even though AltaVista is not specifically medical, it often finds resources that others miss.

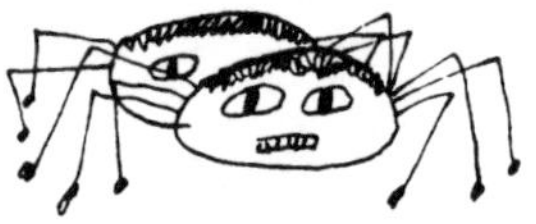

SPIDERS

Spiders, Crawlers, Bots, and Worms

Because there is no physical place where all Internet documents are stored—the information is distributed on machines around the world—a way had to be devised for a computer to compile a database about Web pages. Unbeknownst to most of us, there are a multitude of virtual fuzzies wandering the further reaches of cyberspace on our behalf. The anarchy of the Net made them necessary.

Search engines periodically send these programs (called spiders, web-crawlers, bots, agents, or worms) onto the Internet to look for new Web pages. A bot may send back different pieces of information about a page: title, address, keywords, or even the entire text. This information is then added to a huge index, or database, that the search engine maintains.

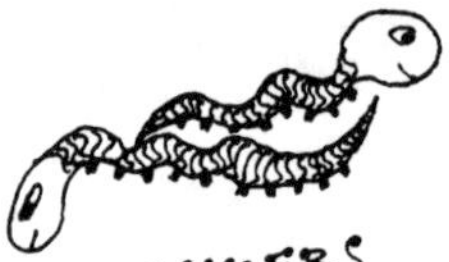

CRAWLERS

Full-Text Search

A full-text search includes all the words in a document or site. For example, if I have the word "Xanadu" in this paragraph, a full-text search will find it. But note that for a person looking for the easy life, finding this paragraph doesn't help: the topic isn't Xanadu at all. In other words, a full-text index will find sites that are irrelevant.

AltaVista indexes all the words in the documents of a site, allowing a full-text search. A comparable medical search engine is Medical World (http://pride-sun.poly.edu), which downloads and indexes the full-text of major medical Internet sites. Because Medical World looks through full-text, it can search for more obscure words; but since it is limited to major medical sites, it will miss smaller or more unusual Web sites.

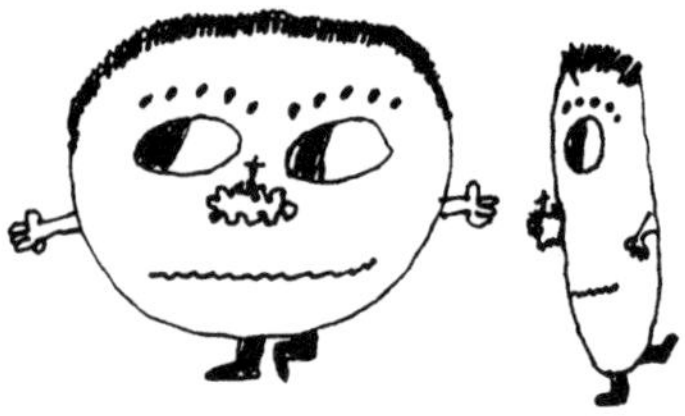

BOTS

The more specific the search words, the more focused the results will be. A search in AltaVista for "travel" gave me five million pages, whereas a search on "Eurorail" found two hundred. Don't use common words such as "and" or "the." (Unless you are specifically using AND, OR or NOT as a Boolean connector; see the next chapter.)

Title or Keyword Search

The indices for some directories are limited to the title or address (URL) of a site. If a word is not part of a title or address, a search will not get any results. Search engines such as these work best with general terms ("trauma") rather than specific ones.

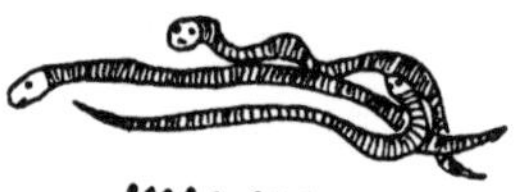

WORMS

Ranking

Most search engines show results in order of the best matches first; in other words, the list of sites will be ranked by how relevant the pages are. Some search engines can show their results in other ways. Excite, for example, has a "View by Web site" link which groups all results from one site together. Sometimes ten or twenty results are simply different documents on the same site; in that case it is better to go to the top-level for the site and look around.

Logical Connectors

This important topic is covered in the next chapter (MEDLINE and CINAHL), but the concepts and techniques apply to general search engines as well.

Searching for a Phrase

Often it is better to search for a phrase ("total joint replacement") rather than a single word. Search engines differ in the way they work with phrases, but most of them will work well with a short phrase ("transient ischemic attack"), and at the top of the results list will be sites where all the words occur together.

Case-sensitive

A search which takes into account capital versus lower-case letters.

Case Sensitivity

The word "case" refers to whether a letter is CAPITALIZED (upper-case) or not (lower-case). If you choose to make a search case-sensitive, that means it will look for the case as well as the word. For example, a case-sensitive search for the word "Paris" will not find "paris." ***Most search engines are set to ignore capitalization if the word is typed in lower case; but if it is typed with a capital letter, they will only look for examples of that word which are capitalized.***

Exact Match

Some search engines and many library search sites have an exact match function. This can be very handy, especially when looking for books, people, places, or other named things. Searching for the exact title "The People's Book of Medical Tests" will be more precise than searching for any of these words individually.

Truncation and Wild Cards

Most search engines include "wild card" characters, which can stand for one letter or several letters. The most common is the asterisk (*). For example, searching for "nurs*" will find matches for nurse, nursing, nursery, even nursoy. Using wild cards often gives too many results, but occasionally the technique comes in handy.

Proximity Search

You may be interested in looking for words that appear in the same sentence or paragraph, but not necessarily in the same phrase. Lycos (http://www.lycos.com) allows you to specify whether words appear NEAR one another; for example, searching for "lincoln near automobile" retrieves pages that talk about a brand of car, rather than the American President.

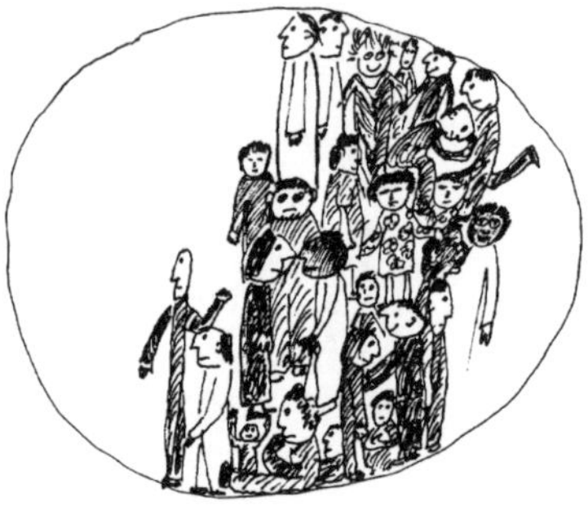

Metasearch

A search engine looks through its own database. Some Web sites, such as Sleuth or Search.com, have a form which sends a search word to several databases. Because more than one site is involved, this kind of search may take longer, but it may also give more results with hard-to-find terms.

Bookmarking a Search

A bookmark can be saved to a search itself, so that it includes the word, phrase, or other parameters. To do this, go to the search engine, type in the words, and run the search. When the results page comes up, add the bookmark.

When you use the bookmark, the engine will re-do the search. This technique is especially useful for information that changes periodically, such as news stories.

Future Developments

So far we have been talking about organization and methods of searching for text documents, but information exists in many other forms: photographs, drawings, wave-forms, radiology images, video, sound. Is it possible for a computer program to automatically index a library of photographs, so that one could search for "automobile" and find all photos that have an auto in them? Or search a library of radiology images for specific abnormalities?

The answer is: soon. For a brief look at these developments, see the article by David Forsyth in the June 1997 issue of *Scientific American*.

> Put all your bookmarks to search engines in a single folder so they will be easy to find.

Points to Remember

Find one or two search engines that meet your needs, then learn how to use them well. Every once in a while re-visit the help file for the search engine, to learn about new features.

Librarians are often the best resource. (After all, they are the consummate "information professionals.") There may be entire types of information that you haven't thought of (support organizations? videotapes? slide collections? reference books? people?).

Becoming an Expert

It's not hard to become reasonably skilled at finding information on the Internet. Here are some simple steps to follow.

Preparation

1. Visit all the major search engines briefly and run a simple search. Bookmark each and organize the bookmarks into folders. Pick one or two and explore advanced options, such as how they handle phrases, truncation, and Boolean logic.
2. Do the same for your medical specialty or any other area of interest.

Doing a Search

1. Before doing a search, spend a minute preparing.
   a) What keywords would best find this topic?
   b) What kind of information is wanted: article? Web site? person to contact?
   c) How urgently are the results needed? Next 24 hours? By the end of the month?
2. Run your search. Skim the list of results looking for a site that matches your needs. Go to that site and look around.
3. Look for lists of links. The links on special-interest sites often provide the best information.
4. When you find what you need, stop to think if you may need to do this search again. If so, bookmark the sites or the search itself.

Reporting the Information

1. Once you find what you need, copy important information to a word processor document for reference. Include the URL of the site!
2. Take a minute to mentally summarize the information.
3. Put the summary into a report, or call/email the person who asked for the search. Tell her how you found it, give her your brief summary, and offer the URL of the site so she can get more details.

For further information on searching, read *Web Search Strategies* (1996, Bryan Pfaffenberger). Or visit http://www.lib.berkeley.edu/TeachingLib/Guides/Internet/FindInfo.html

Search Engines (Medical)

(Links available at http://NewWindPub.com/workbook)

Name/Address	Looks at	Notes
HealthExplorer http://www.healthexplorer.com	database of medical sites	Over 3,000 sites, reviewed.
Health on Net http://www.hon.ch	database of medical sites; reviewed and unreviewed sites.	Database updated by a robot; Uses a thesaurus of medical terms to find Web documents. Sites are rated. Keywords link to related sites. Asterisk (*) acts as wild card.
Medical Search Engines http://phaxp1.gsph.pitt.edu/ Med_Search_Engines.html	several medical search engines	Short descriptions of each engine.
Medical World http://pride-sun.poly.edu	full text of downloaded medical sites	Excellent medical search engine. Uses medical thesaurus; can add terms from this after a search. Can recall searches if you register (free). Can add Boolean logic, but is confusing to use.
Medis http://www.docnet.org.uk/ medisn/searchs.html	journal articles and abstracts	Results include full text or abstract, and journal name. Can have articles emailed to you. Simple search page. Boolean option easy to use. Database limited to traditional medical journals.
Stanford Medbot http://www.med.stanford.edu/ medworld/medbot	up to four search engines	Includes a couple of dozen general, medical, news, and education search engines. Results from each come up in a different frame.

Search Engines (General)

AltaVista http://www.altavista.digital.com	entire Web; Usenet	General search engine, but useful for medical searches. Use quotes for phrases: "unstable angina" Use plus (+) to require a word; minus (-) to exclude it. Advanced search form with Boolean logic.
Excite http://www.excite.com	entire Web	Reviews and ratings of sites. Works better if you enter more words, because of its conceptual indexing. Links to "More like this" next to each result. Plus (+) sign to require a word; minus (-) to exclude it. "View by Web site" groups all results from one site together.

Search Engines (General) *(continued)*

HotBot http://www.hotbot.com	entire Web	Easier than most. Form uses common words for Boolean choices. Buttons along the left limit the search (modify, date, location).
Lycos http://www.lycos.com	entire Web	Advanced "custom" search page with Boolean logic.
Metacrawler http://www.metacrawler.com	entire Web/metasearch	Powerful: searches several engines (AltaVista, Lycos, Excite, etc.) and eliminates duplicate entries.
Savvy Search http://rampal.cs.colostate.edu:200	metasearch	Friendly form. Advanced page can look for people, software, images, news, etc.
Search.com http://www.search.com	metasearch page	Go to Health area. Advanced search page. Plus sign (+) to require a word; minus sign (-) to exclude it. Use quotes for phrases: "unstable angina".
Sleuth http://www.isleuth.com/heal.html	multiple medical engines listed	Metasearch site; links to dozens of medical engines. Can search six at once. Sub-sections: dentistry, diseases, medicine, mental health.

White Pages and Yellow Pages

These sites are continually changing or adding new services.

Bigfoot	http://www.bigfoot.com	Email, telephone, white pages directories. Available in five languages.
Four 11	http://www.four11.com	Email, telephone, yellow pages, government. Available in English, French, Italian.
Knowbot	http://info.cnri.reston.va.us/kis.html	Email, telephone, address.
Infospace	http://www.infospace.com	Email, telephone, address, yellow pages, government, city, and business information.
Internet Address Finder	http://www.iaf.net	Email address.
Internet Sleuth	http://www.isleuth.com/peop.shtml	Metasearch. Links to sites listed in this table.
Lycos People Find	http://www.lycos.com/pplfndr.html	Email, telephone, address, map of address, written directions.
Switchboard	http://www.switchboard.com	White pages, yellow pages.
Yahoo People	http://www.yahoo.com/search/people	Email, telephone, email, home page.

EXERCISES

Each lettered exercise is independent.
(Links available at http://NewWindPub.com/workbook)

I. Guided Practice

A. SEARCH EXCITE

1. Start Netscape or Explorer..
2. Go to http://www.excite.com
3. (Add a bookmark).
4. Click once in the box beneath "Excite Search"
5. Type `dysphagia`
6. Click the Search button or press the Enter key.
7. Find the Dysphagia Resource Center. Click it to go there.
8. Click the Back button to see your search results again.
9. Click View by Web Site. This will group all the results from each site together.

B. SEARCH MEDICAL WORLD

1. Go to http://pride-sun.poly.edu
2. (Add a bookmark).
3. Click once in the text box.
4. Type `dysphagia`
5. Click the Search button or press the Enter key.
6. Note that many of the sites are different from the previous search. The search is limited to major medical Web sites rather than looking through the entire Web.
7. Click a link to the Virtual Hospital. Scroll down.
8. Click on Home at the bottom of the page. In this way you found the Virtual Hospital through a search.

C. SEARCH CLINIWEB

1. Go to http://www.ohsu.edu/cliniweb/search.html
2. (Add a bookmark).
3. Click once in the text box. Type `cancer`
4. Click Submit Query or press the Enter key.
5. Note that there are no results. CliniWeb does better with more terms.
6. Click the Back button.
7. Type all of these words: `cancer leukemia`
`chemotherapy`
`t-cell`
8. Click Submit Query or press the Enter key.
9. Note that you get categories rather than individual links. Select a category and click it.
10. Click on any article.

BROWSE MESH CATEGORIES IN CLINIWEB

1. Scroll to the top of the page.
2. Click Browse in the navigation bar (Browse, Search, Help, Feedback).
3. Click Diseases, then Bacterial and Fungal Diseases, then Bacterial Infections.
4. Take a look at the article on Prevention of Bacterial Endocarditis from the American Heart Association.

D. SEARCH MEDIS

Medis catalogs articles from major medical journals and sites, so the results are limited but of high clinical quality.

1. Go to http://www.docnet.org.uk/medisn/searchs.html
2. (Add a bookmark).
3. In the text box, type `craniofacial`
4. Click the circle with the word Search, or press the Enter key.
5. Click crouzon. Click a link to examine a photo.

E. SEARCH HEALTH ON THE NET

1. Go to http://www.hon.ch
2. (Add a bookmark).
3. In the text box, type `cerebral palsy`
4. Click the Submit button or press the Enter key.
5. Note that there are both reviewed and unreviewed sites listed.
6. Note the keyword links. If you click one of these it will bring up all pages which have that word as a keyword.
7. Scroll down to the bottom of the page. Click Advanced Search.
8. Click in the circular radio button to the left of the word Adjacent. This means that it will look for words you type if they occur in the same sentence.
9. Type `heart attack`
10. Click Submit or press the Enter key.

F. SEARCH ALTAVISTA

1. Go to http://www.altavista.digital.com
2. (Add a bookmark).
3. In the text box, type the following (with the quotation marks): `"supraventricular tachycardia"`
4. Click Submit or press the Enter key.
5. The quotation marks force AltaVista to treat the words as a phrase, rather than looking for each separately.
6. Click Advanced at the top of the AltaVista page.
7. In the first text box, type `intrathecal near narcotic`
8. Click Submit Advanced Query or press the Enter key.
9. This looks for the two words if they occur within ten words of each other on a Web page.

G. SEARCH METACRAWLER

1. Go to http://www.metacrawler.com
2. (Add a bookmark).
3. In the text box, type `fluid and electrolyte balance`
4. Click Search.
5. Watch how it compiles results.
6. Scroll down to take a look at the results.
7. Click Netscape's Back button to return to search page.
8. Click Power Search interface.
9. Select 30 Results per page, 30 Results per source, and timeout of 2 minutes.
10. Click Go.
11. Scroll down and compare these results to your previous search.

II. Problem-Solving

- For neonatology, find a journal, Web site, mailing list, newsgroup, article, drip rates for pressors, ET tube sizes, and a patient handout.
- For stereotactic ventral pallidotomy , find a description of the procedure for the layperson, a list of hospitals where it is done, and the name and email address of a neurosurgeon who performs the surgery.
- Find an email list, newsgroup, Web site, forum, national organization, program of study, and peer reviewed journal for nurse practitioners.
- Choose one medical and one general search engine. On each site run a search on myocardial infarction, then on heart attack. Compare the results from these four searches.

III. Thought and Discussion

- Compare the way you find a house you visited only once; a book in a public library; a resident physician whose name you don't remember; and the staffing ratio for your unit.
- How can a Web site "trick" a search engine into listing it more often, or higher up on a results page?
- Is it possible to design a search engine to find elements inside a picture (e.g. CT scan) or a video (e.g. sleep study)?
- How much of your time at work is spent searching for information? Searching for supplies?

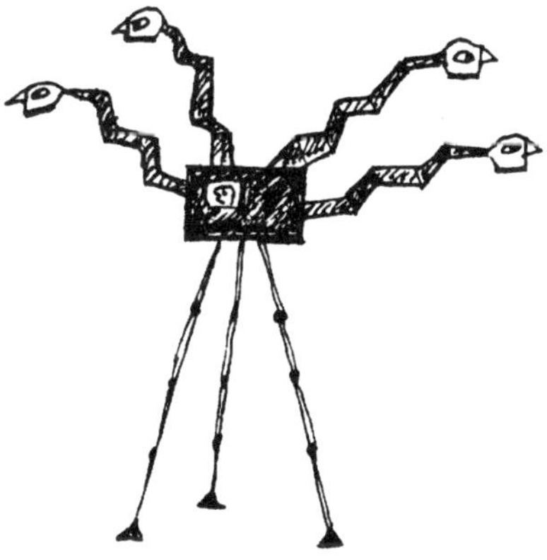

Readings From the Net

(Links available at http://NewWindPub.com/workbook)

Evaluating Search Engines

Eureka	http://www.best.com/~mentorms/eureka.htm	Reviews, form for searching, link to each site and help page for three dozen search engines.
Finding Information on the Internet	http://www.lib.berkeley.edu/TeachingLib/Guides/Internet/FindInfo.html	Most complete tutorial available. Highly recommended.
Finding Information on the Web	http://www.mcp.com/que/et/se_net3/netch3.htm	Chapter from Que book. Detailed instructions for major search engines.
Finding Tools	http://lib-www.ucr.edu/pubs/navigato.html	Long discussion, evaluations, links.
Hints and Tips for Searching the Net	http://www.classroom.net/classroom/searchingfaq.html	Succinct. Includes a troubleshooting guide.
Internet Search Tools	http://www.mtm.kuleuven.ac.be/Services/search.html	Listing, links, and ratings of directories, search engines.
Search Engines	http://www.cnet.com/Content/Reviews/Compare/Search/	Intro, review of ten engines and ten meta-engines.
Search Engine Secrets of the Pros	http://www.zdnet.com/pccomp/features/fea1096/sub2.html	Description and comparison of major general search engines and a short tutorial on Boolean logic from Ziff-Davis, a major computer publisher.
Searching the Internet	http://www.hamline.edu/library/bush/handouts/comparisons.html	Pointers to different documents that discuss search engines.
Search the Net in Style	http://www.cnet.com/Resources/Tech/Advisers/Search	Complete discussion, broken into topics.
Search Tools	http://www.screen.com/start/guide/searchengines.html	Links, tips, documents.
Tips On Popular Search Engines	http://www.hamline.edu/library/bush/handouts/slahandout.html	Quick description and how-to for AltaVista, Excite, Lycos, InfoSeek, WebCrawler, and Yahoo.

Chapter 9: MEDLINE and CINAHL

Some books are to be tasted, others to be swallowed,
and some few to be chewed and digested...

Francis Bacon

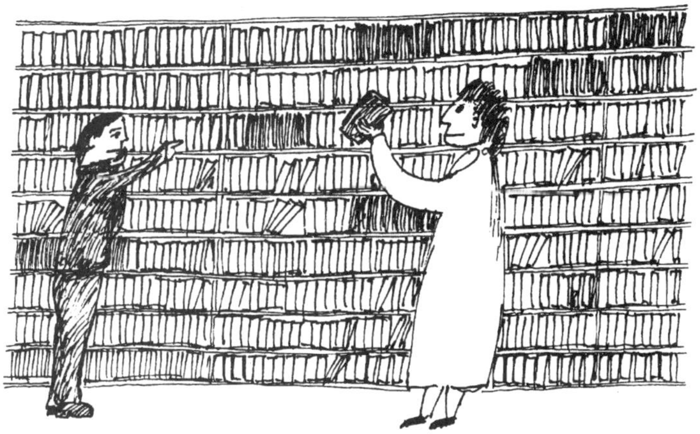

IN THIS CHAPTER

abstract
article type
browsing
catalog
CINAHL
citation
controlled vocabulary
display options
document delivery service
exact matches
field
identifier
MEDLARS
MEDLINE
MeSH
record
reference
save set (save)
subset

MEDLINE versus CINAHL

MEDLINE and CINAHL are the two premier sources, respectively, for citations on medical and nursing literature. Both are indexes to literature for finding citations and abstracts to journal articles. Both are available in print and electronic form. Both allow searches by subject, author, or title; and with both, searches can be modified in various ways. If you need a source for morning rounds in half an hour, you've come to the right chapter.

A bibliographic index is like an extended card catalog: it includes author, title, and journal, and other information such as a short summary (abstract) of the article. Both MEDLINE and CINAHL use a specialized vocabulary, called MeSH, to categorize and organize their indexes.

There are many other, more specialized bibliographic databases available, both in print and electronic form. The best way to find them is usually to go to a special-interest site for a particular specialty. (See Chapter 12 for a directory of such sites.)

Overview of CINAHL

CINAHL (*Cumulative Index to Nursing and Allied Health Literature*) is produced by CINAHL Information Systems (http://www.cinahl.com). It began as a project in the 1940's, and its first official publication was in 1961. In 1984 CINAHL went online, and in 1989 it was released on CD-ROM. Finally, in 1995 it became available directly to individuals via the Internet. All of these are fee-for-service; at the present time CINAHL is not available for free on the Internet. However, access is often available through a school or hospital. The University of California plans to make CINAHL available online to all its campuses.

CINAHL uses about 9,000 terms to index approximately 1,000 nursing and allied health journals going back to 1982. The total number of articles in the database is more than 250,000. About half of these citations have abstracts. CINAHL focuses on issues and materials that are of specific interest to nurses and allied health professionals, and so is an essential tool for nurses who want to do research. It has searchable categories for publication types such as accreditation, CEU, teaching material, nursing diagnosis, nursing intervention, pictorial, clinical path, nurse practice acts, and standards of practice.

CINAHL includes a document delivery service by fax or mail. This means that, for a fee, any article in CINAHL can be obtained.

MEDLINE and the National Library of Medicine

The catalog for the National Library of Medicine (NLM) is called *Index Medicus*; it is a monthly print listing of references to current articles from over 3,100 journals. The *Index Medicus* comes as three separate series of books: author, title, and subject.

In 1966 the NLM put this index on a computerized database called MEDLARS (Medical Literature Analysis and Retrieval System) and made it available to medical libraries. The primary database is called MEDLINE, but there are approximately forty specialized databases, such as AIDSLINE, TOXLINE, and CANCERLIT.

Beginning in 1986 the NLM provided online access to the MEDLARS databases through a program called Grateful Med. (Who thought that up?) Then in April 1996 an Internet version was released so that researchers could get MEDLINE directly over the Internet. MEDLARS, Grateful Med and Internet Grateful Med are available for a fee.

> ***PubMed***
>
> A Web interface to MEDLINE, created by the National Library of Medicine.

Best of all, the NLM has recently developed a free, experimental version of MEDLINE on the Web, called PubMed (http://www.ncbi.nlm.nih.gov/PubMed). With PubMed you can now search the entire MEDLINE database, using Web-based forms. Other Web sites also offer free MEDLINE; see the table at the end of this chapter.

Overview of MEDLINE

MEDLINE is essentially the online version of *Index Medicus*. It includes the *International Nursing Index*, *Hospital Literature Index*, and *Index to Dental Literature*. Currently MEDLINE indexes approximately 4,000 medical and health journals; about 400,000 new article citations are added each year, and the total number of articles indexed since 1966 is about 8.5 million. It is the most frequently searched database in the world. (The physical collection of documents housed in the NLM itself numbers about five million items.)

MEDLINE is more than just a computer version of the print index. It contains many more subject headings, key words, and other ways to make a search more exact. It also indexes more journals than the print version.

Don't confuse the interface used to search MEDLINE with the database itself. There are many different interfaces (Grateful Med, Internet Grateful Med, PubMed, Ovid, Melvyl, various commercial sites) each of which looks different and which may have different functions.

> *Interface*
>
> The way a computer program is set up to interact with you.

MeSH Terminology

The NLM uses a vocabulary of 17,000 terms (called Medical Subject Headings, or MeSH) to categorize medical literature. In addition to being a standard vocabulary for classification, this also provides a hierarchical structure for searching.

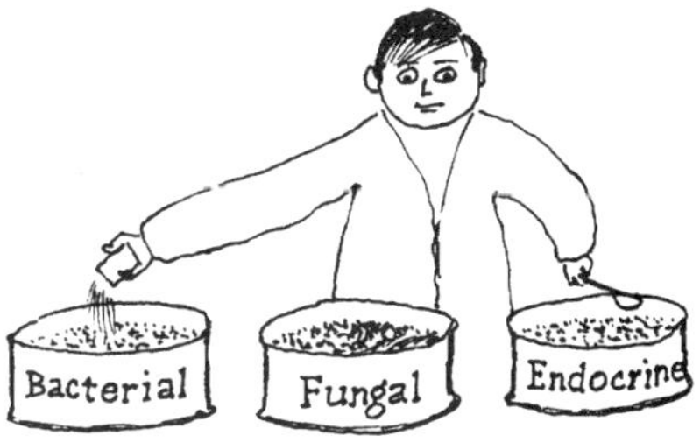

MeSH mush

The top level of MeSH has such categories as anatomy, diseases, or physical sciences. Under diseases are categories for bacterial, fungal, endocrine, immunologic, and so on. Under each of these are subheadings such as diagnosis, etiology, prevention, or therapy.

The classification of medical information is a critical issue, so in 1986 the NLM began a research and development project called the Unified Medical Language System (UMLS) to help integrate medical knowledge. The UMLS contains:

- metathesaurus with information about medical concepts
- lexicon of terms and variation
- semantic network to link the terms in the Metathesaurus
- map of information sources to keep track of such things as bibliographic databases, expert systems, and image databases

For more information about the UMLS, see http://www.nlm.nih.gov/pubs/factsheets/umls.html

What You Find in MEDLINE or CINAHL

MEDLINE and CINAHL are bibliographic databases, in other words, collections of references or citations to articles. A search will retrieve references and abstracts, not the full text of articles.

Shorter articles, such as a letter to the editor or review of a book, will not have an abstract. Abstracts for many non-English journals are available in English, even though the article itself is in a another language. (All abstracts in MEDLINE are written by the author of the article.)

Medical publishers are starting to put the text of their journals on the Internet, but only a small fraction are currently available. For the next few years if you want to get the full text of an article you will have to go to a medical library or use a document delivery service. After that you will probably find the text of most major journals on the Web, though you may have to pay a fee to read or download an issue.

Abstract

A summary of an article.

Some commercial sites, such as HealthGate (http://www.healthgate.com) are connected to document delivery services, so that articles can be ordered immediately. CINAHL has its own document delivery service. The NLM's PubMed site links to publishers who put articles up on the Internet, so that if an article is available online, it is possible to jump directly to it from the citation.

Field

A category in a database.

Search Options

All the information about one article of any database is called a record. A record has different pieces of information; each piece or type of information is called a field. For example, literature databases have fields for title, journal, author, subject, and year of publication. MEDLINE and CINAHL include keywords, language, type of publication (article, letter to the editor, clinical trial), journal subset (nursing, dental literature), and even the age group of patients (infant, child).

When you search for citations you can put in a broad term such as "cancer," or you can limit the search using any of the fields mentioned above. For example, you can look for articles published in 1997 in the journal *Cancer Nursing* with the word "leukemia" in the title.

Searching for a general term often will find thousands of articles, whereas searching for a very specific term or limiting a search too much may give no results at all.

Display Options

Most sites have different ways of displaying the results of a search. The default is often a short form, which will include the author, title, and journal. When you find an article that looks promising, you can then look at the long form or abstract.

Title Word, Key Word, Subject, Abstract?

These are common fields used to search for articles. A subject search on MeSH categories ("subject") is the best place to start if you are looking for a general term, because chances are that MEDLINE has a category for it. For very specific or rare terms, a search by title, keyword or abstract word may get better results.

Logical Connectors: And, Or, And Not

An Internet search site will often present two options: a simple and a complex form for searching. The simple version gives a text box for typing a word or words. The complex version shows many of the fields (subject, publication type) and has more choices.

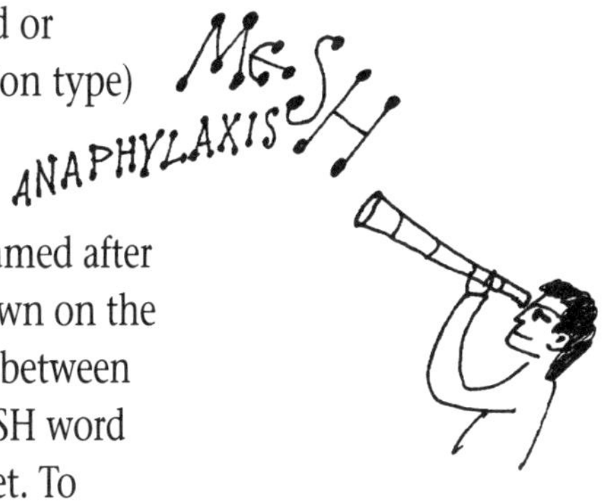

When you search on more than one field, you are using Boolean logic (named after George Boole). Remember set theory in high school, with large circles drawn on the blackboard? Back in 1847 Boole devised a way to work with relationships between words, a kind of algebra for concepts. Suppose that you search for the MeSH word "anaphylaxis" and find 5,000 results. Think of those 5,000 as a group, a set. To make the set smaller, you then modify the search to look for the MeSH term "anaphylaxis" <u>AND</u> title word "antibiotic." The computer will look through the set of 5,000 citations and pull out only those which have the word "antibiotic" in the title. This may give one hundred citations. These hundred are another, smaller set.

"AND" means that both terms must be present. The results for each word constitutes a set; "AND" gives the intersection between those two: a subset of results which contains both words.

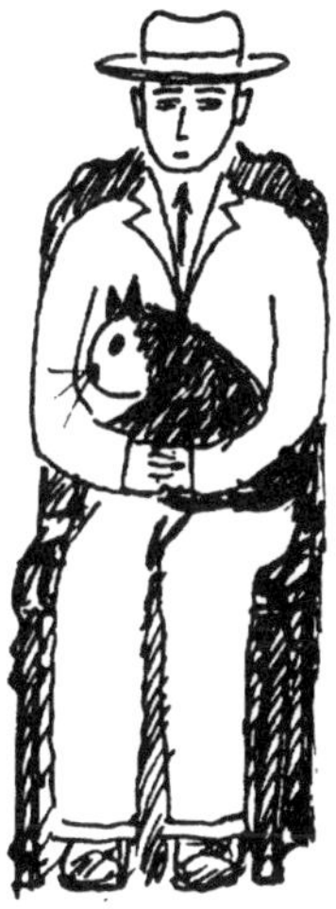

Mr Boole with his cat "Andor"

When evaluating a search with "AND" in a single text box, many search engines will give more weight to the first term, so type the more important term first.

Suppose that searching for the word "antibiotic" results in 20,000 citations, whereas a search for the MeSH word "anaphylaxis" results in 5,000 citations. Searching for title word "antibiotic" <u>OR</u> MeSH word "anaphylaxis," will retrieve 25,000 citations.

"OR" means either/or. You get the union of the two sets: all the results from both. Logical "OR" can be used to expand a search, or make it more inclusive. This is useful for synonyms or different spellings of a word. For example, you can search for "heme OR haeme" so that it finds matches for both the American and British spelling; or search for "kidney OR renal."

> ***Boolean Logic***
>
> The use of the words <u>AND</u>, <u>OR</u>, and <u>NOT</u> to narrow or broaden a search.

Suppose that there are 5,000 citations for the MeSH word "anaphylaxis," and 100 of them have "antibiotic" in the title. Searching for MeSH word "anaphylaxis" <u>AND NOT</u> title word "antibiotic," will retrieve 4,900 citations. It will find the 5,000, but leave out the 100.

By the way, the basic operation of computers, way down there at the micrometer level where electrons are scooting along, is simply Boolean logic: AND, OR, and NOT.

Sets

When you run a search on MEDLINE, it pulls out a subset of the entire database of citations. Several Web sites save the results of each search as a set, then let you to go back and retrieve the results later during the same session. In this way you can revisit a previous search without having to remember all the terms and fields you chose. CINAHL does the same.

Databases on the Net

A database is a structured collection of information, similar to the patient database in a hospital. (See Chapter 17 for a discussion of database programs.) MEDLINE and CINAHL are *bibliographic* or *citation* databases which contain structured information about medical journal articles. On the Internet it is possible to access databases with other kinds of medical information, such as census data, gene information, physicians, medical illustrations, or ICD-9 codes. A database typically has some method of searching, and the techniques and concepts from Chapter 8 will generally apply to a database as well as a search engine.

However, on the Web the word "database" is used loosely for almost any collection of information. A site that claims to have a skin cancer database may in fact have only three handouts, or perhaps a page of links, and there is no way to know (without reading a review of the site) what is there.

Throughout this book are examples of databases:

Chapter 10	Combined Health Information Database
Chapter 12	Gold Multimedia Pharmacy database
Chapter 14	Liszt database of mailing lists and newsgroups
Chapter 16	Microsoft Knowledge Base for troubleshooting

The way to find a database is the same as finding anything else: by subject. If you look for information on AIDS, for example, you will come across several databases; the same is now true for almost every specialty. A few examples of medical databases are given in a table at the end of this chapter.

EXERCISES

Each lettered exercise is independent.
(Links available at http://NewWindPub.com/workbook)

I. Guided Practice

MEDLINE

A. SEARCH THE NLM'S MEDLINE

1. Start Netscape or Explorer.
2. Go to http://www.ncbi.nlm.nih.gov/PubMed/medline.html
3. (Add a bookmark).
4. In the text box type `hantavirus`
5. Click Search or press the Enter key.
6. Click the gray bar Retrieve X documents.
7. The results you see are in citation format. Note the line "citations 1-X displayed..." This tells you how many results there are.

SHOWING ABSTRACTS

1. In the text box to the right of Display, click Citation Report and select Abstract. Then click Display.
2. This will display title and abstract (if there is one) for each article. Scroll down to see the abstracts.

FIND RELATED ARTICLES

1. Click the box Related Articles above any article to see citations similar to that one.
2. This is an extremely powerful function. The NLM uses a formula to compare all the text and MeSH words for an article, and compares these to other articles. The best matches are saved and can be seen by clicking Related Articles. If you find an article that seems to be what you are looking for, the Related Articles will be in effect an instant literature search.

HELP

1. Click the question mark (?) on the navigation banner at the top.
2. This is a 13-page help document that can be printed out.

ADVANCED SEARCH

1. Click the Back button until you are at the first search page.

FIELDS

1. Click All Fields. The list that pops up are fields that you can search. You can search for an author's name, a word in the title, and so on.
2. Select MeSH Terms.

LISTING TERMS FOR A FIELD

1. In the next box, click Automatic and select List Terms.
2. Double-click hantavirus, type `thora` in the text box and click Search, or press the Enter key.
3. When the result page appears, scroll down and look at the text box below "Available terms..." This has MeSH terms that start with thora
4. Next to each term is the number of article citations associated with it. Click thoracic arteries and click Select.
5. Click the gray button which says Retrieve ...Documents to see the citations.

ADD TERMS TO YOUR SEARCH

1. Click Netscape's Back button.
2. In the section "Add Term(s) to Query" click All Fields and select Title Word.
3. Click List Terms and select Automatic. This means it will not give a list of possibilities, but simply add your word to the search.
4. Click to the right of "thoracic arteries," backspace to erase both words, and type `dissection`.
5. Click the Search button.
6. At the top of the result page a line should read: thoracic aorta [MESH] & dissection [TITL]
7. This means that you have searched for the MeSH term "thoracic aorta" AND the title word "dissection" in the Boolean sense of the word AND.
8. In this way you can keep adding terms to a search in order to narrow the results.

SEARCH FOR A PHRASE

1. Click the Clear All link.
2. The search field returns to "All Fields" and the search mode to "Automatic"
3. In the text box type `pulmonary bypass surgery`.
4. Click Search or press the Enter key.
5. You will have more than a thousand results.

PUBLICATION TYPES

1. In the search field, select Publication Type.
2. In the text box, type `review`.
3. Click Search or press the Enter key.
4. The results should be significantly reduced. You have limited the type of article to a review article. Other choices are clinical trial, editorial, interview, letter, monograph, practice guideline, review literature.
5. To see the different publication types, select List Terms in the search mode, type the letter A in the text box, and click Search.

MODIFY THE SEARCH

1. Scroll down to the bottom of the search page.
2. Click pulmonary, then hold down the Ctrl key and click surgery.
3. Let go of the Ctrl key.
4. Click the Search button.
5. Now you have modified the search to pulmonary AND surgery.

START A NEW SEARCH

1. To start a new search, click the Clear All link halfway down the page.

SEARCH FOR ALL TERMS THAT START WITH A GIVEN SET OF LETTERS

1. Click Clear All.
2. Choose Title Word for search field.
3. In the text box, type `fibromy*`
4. (Make sure the asterisk (*) is there.)
5. Click Search or press the Enter key.
6. This retrieves all article citations with words that begin with "fibromy" such as fibromyositis, fibromyoma, or fibromyotomy.

CINAHL

B. SEARCH THE CINAHL DATABASE

1. Start CINAHL. (Requires Ovid CD-ROM)
2. If there is a list, select CINAHL and click OK.

RUN A SEARCH

1. Type `critical paths` and press the Enter key.
2. Critical Paths will be highlighted.
3. Click OK.
4. Click Restrict to Focus. Click OK.
5. Click All Subheadings.
6. Click View, Documents. You will see the first of several hundred documents in a Document Display window. It will show author, institution, journal (source), and subject headings.
7. Along the bottom are buttons. Click Next Doc.
8. Note that your search words are highlighted in red.
9. Note that some articles have abstracts, whereas others don't.

VIEW SHORT FORM (TITLES)

1. Click the Titles button. This gives you a short version for more rapid browsing: Title, author, journal.
2. Click in the scroll bar on the right.
3. Click the Jump To button.
4. Enter the number of an article and click OK.
5. Click the Documents button to see the long form for this citation.
6. Click the Close button to return to the main window.

SEARCH FOR A SPECIFIC JOURNAL

1. Click the Journal button.
2. Type `neo` and press the Enter key.
3. You will see a list of journals.
4. Click Neonatal Network Journal of..., then click OK.
5. Click the line with Neonatal Network.

LIMIT RESULTS TO A TYPE OF ARTICLE

1. Click the Limit Set button.
2. Click Publication Types, then click the Apply button.
3. Scroll through the list. These are types of articles that you can limit your search results to.
4. Click Care Plans, then OK.
5. A window will pop up "Limit Result Set"..."X documents posted in set Y", where X is the number of articles that have care plans, and 2 shows that this is your second search.
6. Click OK, then click Close.
7. Double-click the last line, "Limit X to care plan," to see the documents.
8. Click the Close button to close the document display and return to the main Ovid screen.

SAVE RESULTS TO A FILE

1. Click the last line, "Limit X to care plan."
2. Click the Save button.
3. Type `care` as a name for your file.
4. Click OK.
5. A window will pop up showing the documents being saved to the hard drive.

6. When it is done, a window will say "Documents have been saved in file: c:\... This is where your file is. You can also save directly to a floppy disk.
7. Click OK.

SAVE THE SEARCH STRATEGY ITSELF

1. Click the last line, "Limit X to care plan."
2. Click the Save button.
3. Click Save strategy..., then click OK.
4. The window will say "The highlighted sets will be saved." Click OK.
5. In Save Name, type `neonate`. Press the Tab key to move to the Comments field.
6. Type `care plans in neonatal network journal.`
7. Note that this will save it temporarily, for 24 hours, unless you click the circular button next to permanent. Click OK.
8. A window will pop up "Strategy has been saved..." Click OK.
9. To re-do your search, click File, Open, Open Strategy.
10. Click the line with your saved strategy, the press the Enter key.

SEARCH THE PERMUTED INDEX

1. Click Tools, Permuted Index.
2. Type `women` and press the Enter key.
3. Double-click Employment of Women.
4. Click the Close button.
5. Note that this search is now listed.

LOOK AT SUBHEADINGS FOR A BROAD SUBJECT

1. Click Tools, Subheadings.
2. Type `pain` in the Subheadings window.
3. Scroll down, click Prevention and Control.
4. Click OK.
5. You now have created a search on the subheading of Prevention and Control, under the broad subject of Pain.

II. Problem-Solving

- Find a review of the literature, published in the current year, related to Sudden Infant Death Syndrome.
- Find a critical pathway for wound care published in a nursing journal.
- Find an article on clinical trials for AIDS using stavudine (d4T).
- While in your medical library, compare the time it takes to find an article by walking the stacks versus using MEDLINE.

III. Thought and Discussion

- Ask three professionals how they keep informed about advances in their field.
- Would it be useful for your department or unit to employ a person in a "knowledge position" for searching and finding information?
- Comparing the relative rates of change in knowledge among the occupations of farming, medicine, and the Internet, what kind of person is likely to succeed at each?
- Is it better to read about advances in your field for a few minutes a day, or sit down with an entire journal once a month? What implications does this have for new information delivery methods being developed on the Internet?

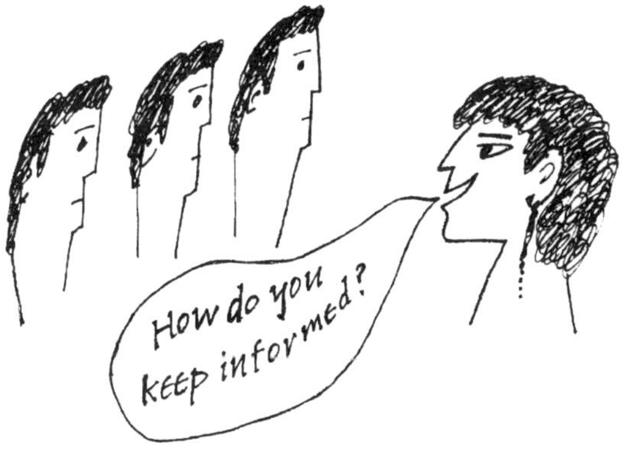

Readings From the Net

(Links available at http://NewWindPub.com/workbook)

MEDLINE and CINAHL

Boolean primer	http://www.cnet.com/Resources/Tech/Advisers/Search/search3.html	Short, practical introduction to the use of Boolean logic in searching the Net.
CINAHL search strategies	http://www.uic.edu/depts/lib/documentation/cinahl.html	A short tutorial covering basic searching of CINAHL.
CINAHL and Ovid	http://www.mcw.edu/lib/ovid_guide.html	Excellent, in-depth explanations.
Evaluating MEDLINE sites	http://avery.med.virginia.edu/~wmd4n/amia/medline.html	Guidelines for evaluating a MEDLINE service, whether free or commercial.
MEDLINE Searching Strategies	http://jeffline.tju.edu/CWIS/OAC/informatics/activities/med_search.html	How to use MEDLINE with OVID. The principles will apply to other ways of using MEDLINE. Very useful if you need help with MeSH, limiting or broadening a search, or the logical connectors AND, OR, AND NOT.
MeSH Headings	gopher://gopher.nlm.nih.gov:70/11/online/mesh	Description of MeSH headings, new headings, new publication types, etc.
MeSH tree	http://www.nlm.nih.gov/mesh	Can get the complete MeSH hierarchy.
Melvyl	http://www.melvyl.ucop.edu	Entry point for Melvyl system. Tutorials and descriptions included.
Quick Guide to MEDLINE Plus	http://www.lib.berkeley.edu/PUBL/medline.html	Tutorial for the command line version of Melvyl's MEDLINE Plus.
Journals Listed in MEDLINE	http://gopher.nlm.nih.gov:70/1/online/journals/lsiou	About four megabytes of files.
Factsheet	http://www.nlm.nih.gov/pubs/factsheets/mesh.html	Factsheet about MeSH, from the NLM.

MEDLINE Sites

Medical Matrix	http://www.medmatrix.org/SPages/Medline.stm	Links to MEDLINE Web sites, with a short description of each site.
MEDLINE Page	http://www.docnet.org.uk/drfelix	Table of sites that provide MEDLINE. Name, coverage, registration (if any), restrictions, delivery services.
Pediatric Points of Interest	http://www.med.jhu.edu/peds/neonatology/medline.html	Table of sites that provide MEDLINE.
National Library of Medicine	http://www.ncbi.nlm.nih.gov/PubMed	Web site provided by the National Library of Medicine for searching MEDLINE.
Community of Science	http://muscat.gdb.org/repos/medl	Collaborative project between Johns Hopkins, others. Subscription based.
Document delivery services	http://www.lib.montana.edu/ILL/docdel.html	Lists and links to different document delivery services.
CarlWeb document delivery service	http://www.carl.org/carlweb	Free searching. Delivery service (UnCover) costs $10 per article by fax.

Miscellaneous Medical Databases

AIDS Patents	http://app.cnidr.org	Twenty years of patents relating to AIDS.
Autopsies	http://www.med.jhu.edu/pathology/iad.html	50,000 autopsy facesheets, 5,000 images.
CDC Wonder	http://wonder.cdc.gov	Huge database of public health data.
Clinical Trials	http://www.centerwatch.com	Several thousand. Email notification service.
ICD-9 and DRG codes	http://www-informatics.ucdmc.ucdavis.edu/icd9/refs.htm	Searchable list.
Mendelian Inheritance	http://www3.ncbi.nlm.nih.gov/Omim	Human genes and genetic disorders.
Rare Disorders	http://myadvisor.com/nord/db/dbsearch/search.htm	Over 1,100 rare diseases.
Physician Directory	http://medseek.com/specsear.stm	Search by specialty, city, or state.
Street drug slang	http://www.drugs.indiana.edu/slang/home.html	3,000 terms.

Chapter 10: Patient Education

I do not believe the patient can be found so demented as to be insensible to the voice of kindness, and the influence of affection upon some of them is really wonderful.

Alice Bennett, MD (1883)

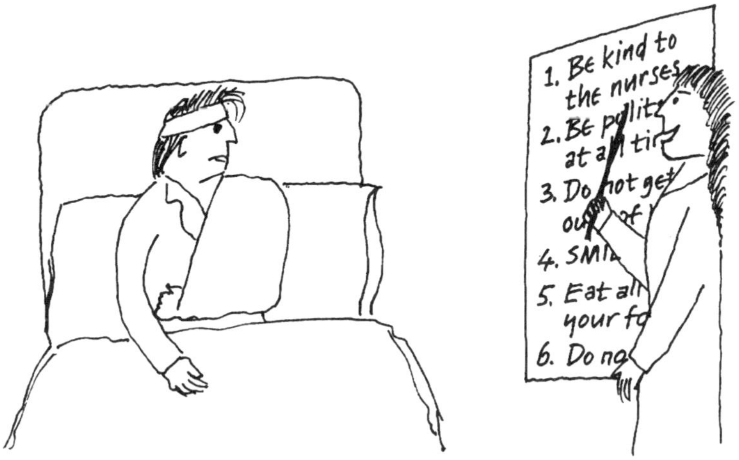
1. Be kind to the nurses
2. Be polit at al tir
3. Do not ge ou of
4. SMI
5. Eat al your f
6. Do no

IN THIS CHAPTER

advocacy
chat
consultation
consumer health
discussion group
fact sheet
family health
forum
hotline
public health
wellness

Patient education is the heart of health care, yet so often good teaching materials have been difficult to find, costly, or unreadable by the general public.

Not any more. Today thousands of handouts on the Internet are freely available for distribution. Many of these include well-done illustrations, and they are written in general vocabulary. This is just the beginning. In the next five years patient education on the Internet will expand faster than any other single topic within health care.

Professional versus Patient Materials

There is no true dividing line between education for the public and that for health care professionals, just as there is no true distinction between medical and nursing knowledge. Although a general rule of thumb when writing a handout is to use a sixth-grade vocabulary and syntax, this rule can be relaxed somewhat when writing for the Internet. Most of the people using the Internet for the next decade will have a higher educational level than the general public, and they will be actively looking for education about medicine and health. In his book *Spontaneous Healing*, physician Andrew Weil points out that "Successful patients search out possibilities for treatments and cures and follow up every lead they come across."

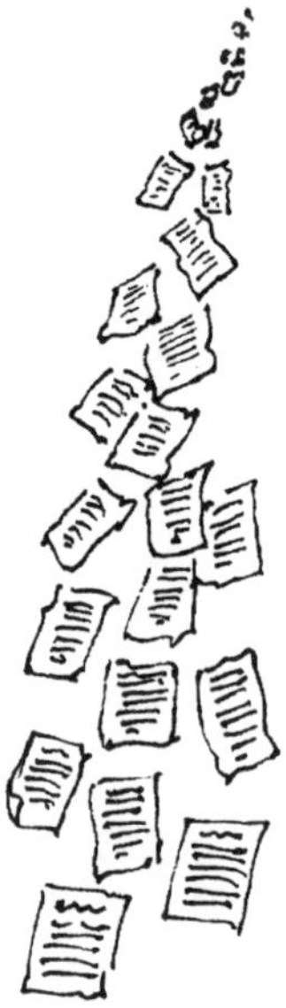

Consumer, Patient, Public, Family Health, Wellness?

Education materials on the Internet are grouped under several categories. Much of what is found in each category is similar, but each of these terms has a specific meaning. Here are the materials generally found in a site or section under these categories:

- Wellness: preventive activities, non-smoking, weight loss, lifestyle changes, diet.
- Family health: pediatrics, childbirth and parenting, infectious diseases, first aid, and care of the elderly.
- Public health: social issues, infectious diseases, pollution, and injuries.
- Patient handouts: disease, hospitalization, procedures, and treatments.
- Consumer health: family health and wellness, consumer rights issues (patient rights, how to choose a physician or HMO).

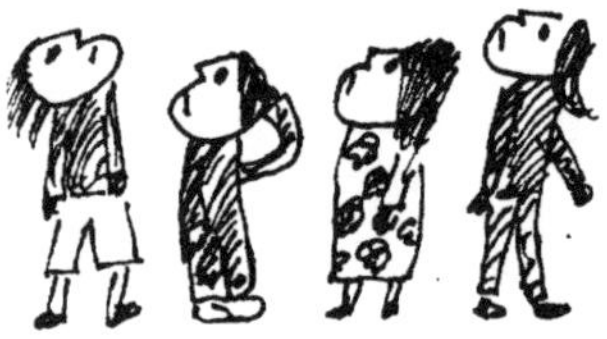

Sites: Governmental, Educational, Commercial, or Individual

It helps to know where a resource is coming from, because that will often determine how freely it can be used. Most government handouts, for example the PDQ series from the National Cancer Institute (http://www.nci.nih.gov), are available for reproduction. Universities and other educational institutions may or may not allow their materials to be copied. Commercial sites, such as MedicineNet (http://www.medicinenet.com), are good sources for information but generally do not want their work reproduced. Individuals who have put up Web sites or who sponsor support groups are often very willing to have their writings copied and used as widely as possible. In every case it is common courtesy to ask permission.

Factsheet, Brochure, Pamphlet, Booklet, Handout?

Most of these distinctions do not apply to educational materials you find on the Internet. A factsheet is usually a short, simple presentation about a limited subject, such as earache or amblyopia, but the same document could be called a brochure or handout. Look at what's in the document, not the category where it is found.

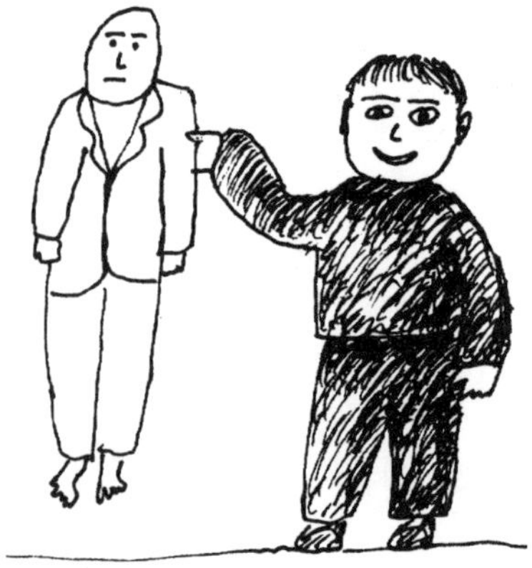

Patient support

Support, Advocacy Consultation

Patient support sites or organizations commonly have educational materials, mailing lists, toll-free numbers, print newsletters, and even national gatherings related to a specific disease or condition. Many of these sites were started by persons with the condition, so they tend to be very open and patient-oriented. Advocacy groups overlap with support groups to a great extent, but advocacy specifically means acting on behalf of another, and a true advocacy organization often fights for increased patient rights.

Web sites offering consultation for the public are still rare. See Chapter 13 for a discussion of the ethical and legal issues regarding direct advice to the public.

Email Lists, Discussion Groups, Hotlines, Forums, Chat

See Chapter 14 for more about email lists and Usenet discussion groups. These are technical protocols on the Internet which use email to post a question or comment to a group.

Forum

A place for (written or verbal) public discussion.

Having the ability to interact with someone is critical for healthcare, because so much of compliance hinges upon the relationship that is set up between patient and provider. "It takes two to speak the truth,—one to speak, and another to hear." (Henry David Thoreau) Different methods are available for patients and providers to interact. A hotline is a phone number to call for information. In the past a forum was a public place where people met to discuss matters, but now it often refers to some kind of discussion group, often conducted through the Usenet. Magazines often have a forum section where people pose questions to one another or to an expert. Chat refers to a site or page where several people can exchange comments back and forth in real-time; it works much like a conference call. In comparison, with a discussion group or email list you post a question and then wait a day or two for answers.

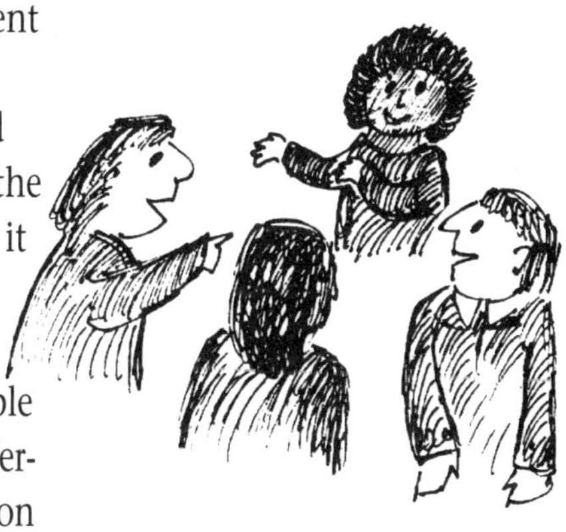

Text and Multimedia

Most of the consumer education materials available on the Internet today are straight text, with a few pictures. This will change rapidly in the next few years, as more people become Web authors and the capacity of the Internet expands to include audio and video.

Internet versus CD-ROM

Several family health encyclopedias are now available on CD-ROM. The J.A. Majors Company (http://www.majors.com) publishes a medical multimedia catalog which covers the entire health care field, not just consumer health. Its spring 1997 version, with about 300 titles, covers every discipline from Administration to Urology.

Popular consumer health CD-ROMs are the ADAM anatomy series (Nine Month Miracle, The Inside Story) and the Mayo series (Family Health Clinic, Family Pharmacist).

EXERCISES

Each lettered exercise is independent.
(Links available at http://NewWindPub.com/workbook)

I. Guided Practice

A. PATIENT EDUCATION: HEALTHFINDER

1. Start Netscape or Explorer..
2. Go to http://www.healthfinder.gov
3. (Add a bookmark).
4. Click Search.
5. Note that you can search alphabetically, or by topic.
6. Scroll down and click arthritis.
7. Click For more details link underneath Coping with Arthritis in its Many Forms.
8. Click the Internet URL (http://www.fda.gov/...) to see the article.
9. Click the Back button.
10. Click the link under Sponsoring Agency (Office of Consumer Affairs...) This takes you to a listing of other sites sponsored by the same agency, with organizational info, contact numbers, description, online resources, and print resources. Very useful.

B. PATIENT SUPPORT: NATIONAL HEALTH INFORMATION CENTER

1. Go to http://nhic-nt.health.org
2. (Add a bookmark).
3. Click the icon with a question mark, or scroll down the page to the section which reads Health Information Resource Database.
4. Click Search the Database for a Particular Entry.
5. Click Title and choose Keyword.
6. Click in the text box next to "The term you..." and type `depression`.
7. Click Start Search or press the Enter key.
8. Click the link for the National Mental Health Association.
9. Note the contact information, link to their home page; abstract; and publications.
10. Scroll down to the Keywords section. You can use these to see a list of resources for related conditions or concepts.
11. Click Suicide to see a list.
12. Click the NHIC Home Page link at the bottom of the page to return to the beginning.

TOLL-FREE NUMBERS

1. Scroll down to the Health Information Resource Database section again.
2. Click Toll-Free Numbers for Health Information.
3. Use Netscape's Find function to see if there is an organization for ostomy patients.
4. Click the Edit, Find menu (Netscape 4: Edit, Find in Page).
5. Type `ostomy` and press the Enter key.
6. Click the Cancel button in the Find window to close it. The United Ostomy Association link should be highlighted.
7. Click the NHIC Home Page link at the bottom of the page to return to the beginning.

KEYWORD LIST OF RESOURCES

1. Scroll down and click the link Search using the Keyword Listing of Resources in the Database.
2. Scroll down. Here is a list of frequently requested topics. Click one to see what is available.

C. PATIENT EDUCATION: MEDHELP

1. Go to http://medhlp.netusa.net
2. (Add a bookmark).
3. Click the Search icon at the top of the page.
4. Click in the text box and type `lupus`
5. Click the Search button.
6. Note the three kinds of resources listed: glossary entries, articles in MedHelp, and articles from other Internet sites.
7. Click the Discoid Lupus Erythematosus link in the section Articles from other Internet sites. You will see a close-up photo of a forearm showing this condition.
8. Note that the MedHelp navigation bar is still visible at the top of the screen. The lupus page is in a separate frame.

GLOSSARY

1. Click the Netscape Back button.
2. Click the second Drug-Induced Lupus entry in the glossary section.
3. In the definition, click thrombocytopenic purpura. This is an excellent example of a hypertext dictionary. The home page is http://www.drschueler.com

PEER REVIEW

1. Click the About link on the MedHelp navigation bar.
2. Click Our Advisory Board or scroll down to this section.
3. Note that they use medical professionals for each field to assure the accuracy of the information on their site.

D. PATIENT EDUCATION: HEALTHANSWERS

1. Go to http://www.healthanswers.com
2. (Add a bookmark).
3. Click Search on the right side of the navigation bar.
4. Click in the text box and type `breast cancer`
5. Click the words Click to get an Answer or press the Enter key.
6. Click Cancer Facts for People Over 50. Note that it is a simple text document.
7. Click Netscape's Back button.
8. Click mammography.
9. The table of contents links take you to sections in this document.
10. Scroll down and click X-ray. This takes you to a document explaining X-rays. Scroll down to the bottom and click barium x-ray to read about barium enema. Note how easily you can move around a hypertext collection of documents this way.

LISTS OF RESOURCES

1. Click the Netscape Back button until you return to the Search page.
2. Click First Aid in the list of Wellness resources.
3. Note that these resources come up in a separate frame. Scroll down to see how HealthAnswers organizes its resources.
4. Click Tests, then Tests and Procedures Index.
5. Scroll down and click BUN.
6. Scroll through the information to see what is available.

II. Problem-Solving

- Find a list of the National Cancer Institute's handouts for the public on treatment information.
- For mental health, find a Web site, hotline, mailing list, local support organization, and news on legislation.
- For someone in your family with a chronic condition, find and print a patient handout from the Internet.

III. Thought and Discussion

- What percentage of the average person's medical information comes from each of these three sources: friends and family; printed material; healthcare providers?
- In terms of treatment outcome, what is the relative importance of the knowledge a patient has about her condition compared to the knowledge of the healthcare provider?
- It is said that ours is a time of "experts" who tell us how we should do everything from raising children to managing our money. How will the Internet affect this?

Guides to Internet Sites With Consumer Information

(Links available at http://NewWindPub.com/workbook)

Guides to Patient Education Sites

HealthWeb	http://www.uic.edu/depts/lib/health/hw/consumer/internet.html	A well-annotated set of links to resources, arranged by disease (aging, AIDS, allergies, etc.).
MedWeb Consumer Health	http://www.gen.emory.edu/MEDWEB/keyword/consumer_health.html	A huge list (over 450 Kb) of consumer health sites. By keyword.
	http://www.gen.emory.edu/MEDWEB/alphakey/consumer_health.html	Same list, alphabetical.
Nashville Health Page	http://www.nashville.com/~Gsnace/health_2.htm	Listing of sites by topic (allergy, arthritis, etc.) No annotations, but each link identifies the source. Links are directly to handouts on each topic.
Patient Education and Support	http://www.medmatrix.org	Medical Matrix lists and reviews sites that provide patient education handouts.
Patient/Consumer Health Information	http://www.kumc.edu/service/dykes/RRPAGES/patient/phmpage.html	Resource provided by Dykes Library at Kansas University Medical Center. The KUMC librarians give a one-paragraph review of each site for content, format and ease of use. Not a very extensive list, but the reviews make it a valuable starting point.

Patient Organizations and Support Groups

American Self-Help Clearinghouse	http://www.cmhc.com/selfhelp	Many different resources for finding a support group (worldwide) or how to start a group. List of online resources, alphabetical by topic (100 topics: abuse, adoption, aging, etc.) with Web sites, mailing lists, and newsgroups. List of mental health resources arranged by symptom (anorexia, bereavement, bipolar).
Health Hotlines	http://www.cdcnac.org/sis	Searchable list from the National Library of Medicine of 17,000 organizations, databases, agencies, telephone hotlines, Web sites, etc.
Health Information Resources	http://nhic-nt.health.org	From the DHHS. Its purpose is to put consumers and professionals in touch with organizations. List of 400 organizations: toll-free numbers, email and Web links (if available). Keyword links to a related list or organization. Links to 65 health-related government centers.
Patient Advocacy Numbers	http://infonet.welch.jhu.edu/advocacy.html	List of 200 support organizations, with toll-free numbers and links to Web pages (currently about 80).
Support Resources	http://www.cmhc.com/sxlist.htm	Part of Mental Health Net (http://www.cmhc.com) which is itself a valuable source of information and resources.

Patient Handouts

Boston Univ. Medical Center	http://web.bu.edu/COHIS	Highly graphic and multimedia collection of copyrighted material on community health topics. You can find resources in a number of ways (searching, browsing, site map).
Combined Health Info Database	http://chid.nih.gov	Citation database, similar to MEDLINE or CINAHL, except specifically for patient handouts. Combination database from the NIH and CDC. Searchable.
HealthAnswers	http://www.healthanswers.com	One-stop commercial site for family health information. Has several different ways to find information: alphabetically, by disease, by symptom, anatomy (eyes, immune system) or by topic. Has a series of handouts from the American Academy of Family Physicians, a hypertext encyclopedia ("knowledge base"), and links to other resources. An excellent resource for the layperson to educate herself about common health questions and conditions.
The Health Explorer	http://www.healthexplorer.com	Commercial site with links to more than 3,000 Web sites. Descriptions and reviews of sites. Search engine and browsable list of topics. In addition to topics such as diseases or nutrition, they have hospitals, health insurance, and physicians. Straightforward and easy to use.
Healthfinder	http://www.healthfinder.gov	U.S. government site providing a gateway for consumer health information from the government. Alphabetical and topic listing. Each resource includes a short review, a long review, and a link to the document.
Healthgate	http://www.healthgate.com	Impressive array of resources, both free and subscription. Also professional sources such as MEDLINE, Cancerlit.
Healthtouch	http://www.healthtouch.com	Commercial site that collects documents from government agencies, formats them for easy viewing and printing, and makes them available. Top page is a topic list (allergy, arthritis, cancer); each topic page has individual handouts. All documents provided by the government, so this is good starting point if you want to build up a set of handouts for a clinic or institution.
HealthWatch	http://www.aetnaushc.com/topics	Series of 75 copyrighted handouts from Aetna US Healthcare, listed alphabetically by topic.
Mayo Health Oasis	http://healthnet.ivi.com	From the Mayo Clinic. Very friendly format.

Patient Handouts *(continued)*

Med Help International	http://medhlp.netusa.net	Excellent. A not-for-profit organization. Has a medical advisory board, a 6,000-word glossary, over 1,000 support groups, forums, and an innovative section that allows patients to get in touch with others who have a similar condition.
MedicineNet	http://www.medicinenet.com	400 copyrighted handouts in common language. Links to related Web sites and references.
NIDDK	http://www.niddk.nih.gov	Diabetes; endocrine and metabolic, hematologic, urologic, and kidney diseases; nutrition and obesity.
Patient Education	http://lib-sh.lsumc.edu/fammed/pted/pted.html	From Louisiana State University Medical Center.
RxMed	http://www.rxmed.com/handouts.html	Handouts on 400 common conditions.
Virtual Hospital	http://vh.radiology.uiowa.edu	The Virtual Hospital from the University of Iowa has a "Health Book" with about 100 copyrighted handouts on disease-related topics. Searchable, or browse by organ system or department.
Wellness Web	http://www.wellweb.com	Women's health, smoking, pain, senior's center, cancer. Dozens of documents.

Online Medical Advice

Sites may take questions and post answers, or email answers privately, or both. Many of these are similar to an advice column in a magazine.

Arthritis Foundation	http://www.arthritis.org	Arthritis
Ask A Doc	http://www.rain.org/~medmall/ask/asklandon.html	Pediatrics
Ask the Doctor	http://www.health-net.com/ask.htm	Any topic
Ask the Pharmacist	http://webmaster.wilmington.net/dees	Pharmacology
Ask Tori, RN	http://www.storksite.com	Pregnancy and childbirth
Breast Cancer Answers	http://sadr.biostat.wisc.edu/bca/ask.html	Breast cancer
Children With Diabetes	http://www.castleweb.com/diabetes	Diabetes
DentistZone	http://www.dentistzone.com	Dentistry
DentistInfo	http://www.dentistinfo.com	Dentistry
Fertilitext	http://www.fertilitext.org	Infertility
LifeTime Online	http://www.lifetimetv.com/parenting/RESOLVE/RESOLVE.HTM	Infertility
Mental Health Infosource	http://www.mhsource.com	Mental health, psychiatry
ParentsPlace.com	http://www.parentsplace.com	Pediatrician, dentist, midwife, lactation consultant, nutritionist
VisionCare	http://www.visioncare.com	Optometry, vision
World Federation of Hemophilia	http://sadr.biostat.wisc.edu/bca/ask.html	Hemophilia

Chapter 11: Medical Journals and News

We should read, not in order to forget ourselves and our daily lives, but on the contrary, in order to gain a firmer, more conscious, more mature grip on our own lives.

Hermann Hesse

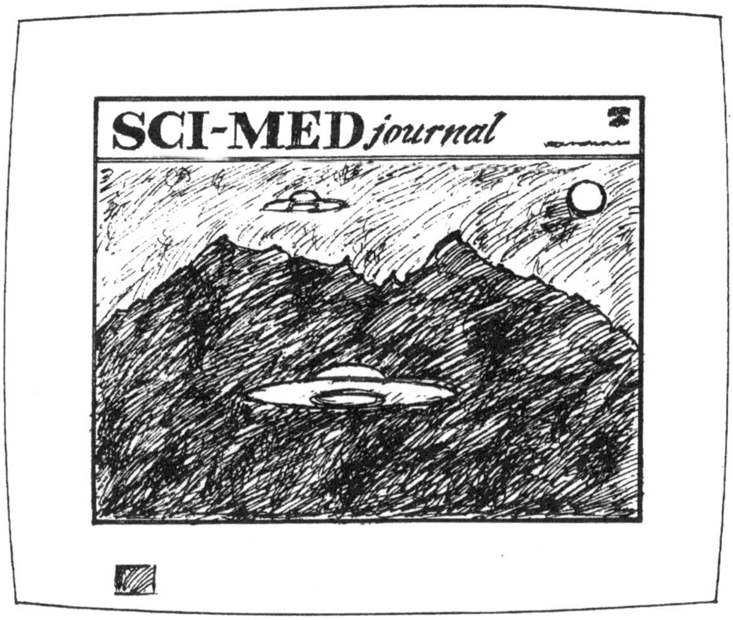

IN THIS CHAPTER

abstract
document delivery service
news service
peer review
table of contents

Current Events

Apart from education and research, every professional needs to stay current with changes in a specialty, whether it is urology or desktop publishing. Periodicals (magazines and newspapers) are one convenient source for current information, and for many professionals their specialty journal is a main source, practically speaking, for continuing education. For general news we increasingly rely upon television.

Traditional Print Media

A traditional journal has an editorial board which reviews each article for style, consistency, and accuracy.

Editors hold themselves to high standards, so each issue is carefully crafted. Money from subscriptions and advertising pays an office staff, and authors are commissioned to write articles. Most importantly, scientific and medical journals generally have a peer-review process whereby each article is submitted to several experts in the same field, who review the content. Traditional journals, in other words, can be trusted to provide authoritative information.

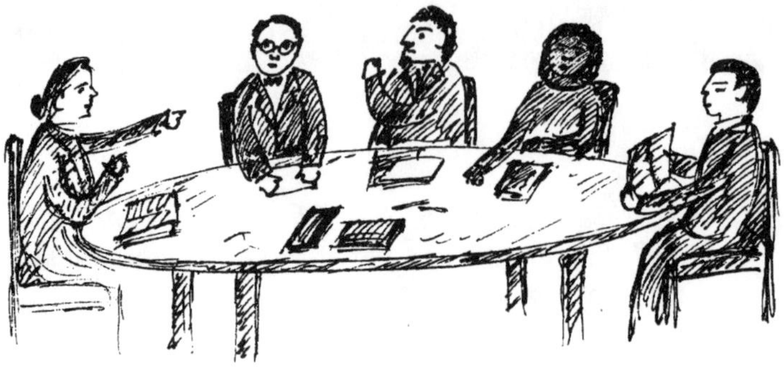

But there are drawbacks to these journals. They are often conservative in their choice of topics, and unwilling to publish articles or opinions which are contrary to the status quo. Although they will deny it, advertising money surely affects the choice of which articles to publish. The turn-around between the time an author first contacts a journal and the publication date is often 9-12 months, which is not practical for a rapidly changing field such as the Internet. Finally, many journals become victims of their own success: as they become established, they restrict themselves to well-known authors and subjects.

Alternatives

Most alternatives to print journals existed long before the Internet, but electronic publishing has accelerated their growth and created new ones. Organizations have newsletters that are published monthly or quarterly, with events, reviews, and other timely information. Journal clubs are used by professionals to talk with others in the same field about the latest research. Conferences often turn out to be invaluable for discovering new and upcoming trends.

The Electronic Revolution

The Internet has changed publishing dramatically. For those who use it, the Internet revolutionizes the process of keeping up with events. News stories are linked to in-depth coverage of related issues, events, and people; a custom news page can be specified so that you get only certain topics; you can have automatic notification for certain Web sites so that you get a message when the site changes. And this is just the beginning.

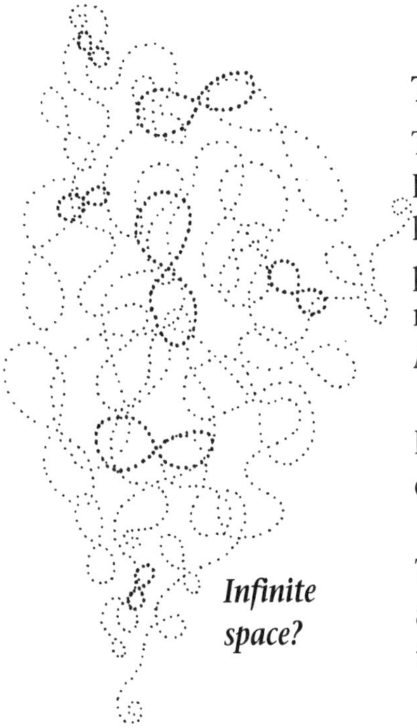

Infinite space?

Internet publishing is instantaneous. The second you put it up, millions of people can read it.

The Internet has infinite space. You can put up issues of a journal for 10 years, and all the issues will be available. No more fumbling through your shelves for that article you read six months ago.

But—anyone can publish. Nothing prevents someone from putting up a home page, calling it The World's Most Important Medical Information, and then writing whatever he pleases. No editor will correct the grammar, nobody will check the facts, no peers will tell him that his research is flawed. Worst of all, those who know nothing about medicine may read it and act upon faulty or incorrect information.

Medical Journals on the Internet

Publishers of medical journals are still worried that they will lose money by making their text available in electronic form, so they have been slow to adopt this new medium. As the exchange of money on the Internet becomes more common, publishers will devise subscription or pay-per-view methods of reading their journals online. Some publishers allow free access to their journal for a trial period, then later require subscription in order to read the online version.

Journals that have "online" in the name usually have the most materials available. They also tend to use more graphics, include online forums for discussing the articles, links to other sites, and in general have a wider spectrum of electronic and Internet tools. Some of these, such as the *Journal of Obstetrics and Gynecology Online* and several others by CCS Publishing, are only published on the Internet and do not appear in paper form. Even so, they adhere to traditional standards of peer review and editing. Other online publications, such as *Cancer Online*, are electronic versions of an existing paper journal.

> ***Online***
>
> Any process that occurs while you are connected to a network, as opposed to working on an isolated computer.

EXERCISES

Each lettered exercise is independent.
(Links available at http://NewWindPub.com/workbook)

I. Guided Practice

A. NEWS: FOR CONSUMERS

1. Go to CNN http://www.cnn.com/HEALTH
2. (Add a bookmark).
3. The page may take a minute to download because it has several graphics.
4. Click Full Story beneath any of the summaries to read the complete article.
5. Scroll down to the bottom of a story. Note that there is a "Related sites" section at the bottom which links to Internet sites with more information on that story.

B. NEWS: SUB-TOPICS

1. Go to http://www.newspage.com
2. (Add a bookmark).
3. Scroll down. Click Healthcare on the left-hand list.
4. Click Medical Equipment, Devices & Supplies.
5. Click Cardiovascular Devices.
6. Click the title of an article to read it.

C. NEWS: LINKED STORIES

1. Go to http://www.lycos.com/health
2. (Add a bookmark).
3. Click Top Story.
4. Look below the summary.
5. Click the link below the line "Get the full story at"
6. This takes you to any one of many Web sites that carry full news stories.

D. JOURNALS: FIND A JOURNAL

1. Go to http://www.hslib.washington.edu/journals
2. (Add a bookmark).
3. Click any letter to see an alphabetical list of journals and links.

E. JOURNALS: ARTICLES BY TOPIC

1. Go to WebMedLit (http://www.webmedlit.com)
2. (Add a bookmark).
3. Note the journal titles along the left side. These are the source of the articles.
4. Click the Immunology topic.
5. Click on a title. Some journals will have full-text articles, others abstracts, and others will require registration. Most of the Archives journals require a (free) registration on the AMA site: (http://www.ama-assn.org)

F. JOURNALS: NURSING ARTICLE SEARCH

This is an article search engine provided by Springhouse Publishing. It looks through 100 different nursing journals.

1. Go to http://www.springnet.com/journals.htm
2. (Add a bookmark).
3. Scroll down. Click Search the Springhouse Reference Library.
4. Scroll down. Click Agree.
5. Click Press to enter the Springhouse Reference Library.
6. Click in the text box and type `clinical pathway`Click Search.
7. Click the Display button.
8. Scroll down to see abstracts and other information on the articles.
9. Use Netscape's Back button to return to the search page.
10. Click to uncheck the Words Anywhere box and click to check the Title box.
11. Click in the text box and type intravenous.
12. Click the Search button.
13. Scroll down. Note the history of your searches at the bottom. You can click one of these to see those records again, or you can merge them using Boolean AND or OR.

G. JOURNALS: AMERICAN MEDICAL ASSOCIATION

Register at the AMA site (free) so you can read abstracts from their journals.

1. Go to http://www.ama-assn.org
2. (Add a bookmark).
3. Click JAMA in the graphic.
4. Click registration.
5. If you wish, fill out the form and submit it to get a login name and password. These will allow you to read the abstracts and other materials on the AMA site.

III. Thought and Discussion

- What makes an online medical journal "authoritative"? See http://www.library.cornell.edu/okuref/research/skil26.htm for one set of criteria in evaluating a source.
- Distinguish between a newsletter, journal, news story, citation, abstract, forum posting, and editorial.
- If you were the editor of an online Web page or newsletter in your field, how would you determine the accuracy of the information that you publish?

Medical News (Directories)

Achoo	http://www.achoo.com/newspage
Ecola Directories	http://www.ecola.com/news/press
Internet Sleuth	http://www.isleuth.com/news.html
Library of Congress	http://lcweb.loc.gov/global/ncp/lists.html
MedWeb	http://www.gen.emory.edu/medweb/medweb.news.html

Medical News (Individual Sites)

AMA News	http://www.ama-assn.org
Cable News Network	http://www.cnn.com/HEALTH
Chic. Tribune	http://www.chicago.tribune.com/articles/n_news
International Medical News	http://www.sma.org/intl/interndx.htm
Lycos	http://www.lycos.com/health
Newspage	http://www.newspage.com
Nursing World	http://www.nursingworld.org/connect.htm
NYT Synd.	http://nytsyn.com/med
Reuters	http://www.reutershealth.com
Science Daily	http://www.sciencedaily.com
The Scientist	http://www.the-scientist.library.upenn.edu
USA Today Health	http://www.usatoday.com/life/health/lhindex.htm

In the table below, I use the following to indicate what is available on a site.

- abstract — abstracts only
- text — some full-text articles
- full journal — complete contents of journal
- subscription — subscription to the site or the journal required to view text
- membership — membership in the professional organization required to view text

Medical and Nursing Journals Online (Summaries and Collections)

(Links available at http://NewWindPub.com/workbook)

BioMedNet	http://biomednet.com	Text of the Current Opinions journals; subscription
Electronic Journals in Health Sciences	http://www.hslib.washington.edu/journals	Alphabetical list, probably the best. Annotations tell you what is available, whether it is a subscription service, etc.
Elec. Newsletters and Journals	http://www.mfhs.edu/library/webinfo/journal.htm	Single alphabetical list. Annotation shows only sponsoring organization.
Electronic Publications	http://www.gen.emory.edu/MEDWEB/alphakey/electronic_publications.html	Alphabetical listing of hundreds of journals. Also a list arranged by category.
Elsevier	http://www.elsevier.nl/catalogue	Dozens of tables of contents.
Kansas Univ.	http://www.kumc.edu/dykes/journals/display.html	Lists online biomedical journals which have at least a table of contents available.
MD Digests	http://php2.silverplatter.com/physicians/digest.htm	Digests of five top journals.
Medis	http://www.docnet.org.uk	Search engine for full-text articles.
Primary Care Reviews	http://www.mcphu.edu/libraries/resources/reviews	Abstracts and reviews categorized by disease and topic; links to journal sites.
Springhouse	http://www.springnet.com/journals.htm	Search facility for 100 nursing journals, with abstracts.
WebMedLit	http://www.webmedlit.com	Links to articles arranged by subject.

Medical Journals

(Links available at http://NewWindPub.com/workbook)
To save space, the word "Journal" is often abbreviated to "J."

Journal	*Address*	*Available*
Aerospace Medicine and Biology	http://www.sti.nasa.gov/Pubs/Aeromed/Aeromed.html	full journal
Aesclepian Chronicles	http://www.forthrt.com/~chronicl/homepage.html	text
AIDS Daily Summary	gopher://cdcnac.org:72/11/2	full journal
AIDS Information Newsletter	gopher://gopher.niaid.nih.gov:70/11/aids/vaain	full journal
AIDS Weekly	http://www.newsfile.com	subscription
Alcohol Alert	http://www.niaaa.nih.gov	full journal
Alternative Medicine Digest	http://www.alternativemedicine.com	full journal
Alzheimer's Disease Review	http://www.coa.uky.edu/ADReview	full journal
American Academy of Orthopedic Surgeons Bulletin	http://www.aaos.org/wordhtml/bulletin.htm	full journal
American Association of Anatomists newsletter	http://www.anatomy.org/anatomy/newshead.html	full journal
American College of Physicians Journal Club	http://www.acponline.org	membership

Journals *(continued)*

American College of Physicians Observer	http://www.acponline.org/journals/news/obstoc.htm	text
American College of Radiology Bulletin	http://www.acr.org	membership
American Gastroenterological News	http://www.gastro.org	full journal
American J. of Anesthesiology	gopher://gasnet.med.yale.edu	abstracts
American J. of Clinical Nutrition	http://www.faseb.org/ajcn	abstracts
American Journal of Health System Pharmacy	http://www.ashp.org	text
American Journal of Nursing	http://www.ajn.org	text
American J. of Ophthalmology	http://www.ajo.com	full journal
American Journal of Pathology	http://journals.at-home.com/PATHOLOGY	abstracts
American Medical News	http://www.ama-assn.org	text
Amyloid	http://med-med1.bu.edu/amyloid/amyloid.html	abstract
American J. of Epidemiology	http://www.sph.jhu.edu/pubs/jepi/default.htm	abstracts
American Psychological Association Monitor	http://www.apa.org/monitor	full journal
Anaesthesia On-line	http://www.priory.com/journals/anaes.htm	full journal
Annals of Internal Medicine	http://www.acponline.org	text
Annals of Thoracic Surgery	http://www.sts.org/annals	full journal
American Journal of Maternal-Child Nursing	http://www.ajn.org/mcn	text
American Journal of Nursing	http://www.ajn.org/ajn	text
Annals of Saudi Medicine	http://www.kfshrc.edu.sa/annals	text
Antimicrobial Agents and Chemotherapy	http://www.asmusa.org/jnlsrc/journal.htm	abstracts
Antiviral Agents Bulletin	http://www.bioinfo.com/biotech/antiviral.html	full journal
Antiviral Weekly	http://www.newsfile.com	abstracts
Applied and Environmental Microbiology	http://asmusa.org/jnlsrc/aem1.htm	abstracts
Archives of Dermatology	http://www.ama-assn.org	text
Archives of Family Medicine	http://www.ama-assn.org	text
Archives of General Psychiatry	http://www.ama-assn.org	text
Archives of Internal Medicine	http://www.ama-assn.org	text
Archives of Ophthalmology	http://www.ama-assn.org	text
Archives of Otolaryngology Head & Neck Surgery	http://www.ama-assn.org	text
Archives of Neurology	http://www.ama-assn.org	text
Archives of Surgery	http://www.ama-assn.org	text
Archives of Pediatrics and Adolescent Medicine	http://www.ama-assn.org	text
Archives J. Club-Women's Health	http://www.ama-assn.org	text
Association for Research in Otolaryngology newsletter	http://www.aro.org	full journal
Australian Elec. Journal of Nursing Education	http://www.csu.edu.au/faculty/health/nurshealth/aejne/aejnehp.htm	full journal
Berkeley Wellness Letter	http://www.enews.com/magazines/ucbwl	text
Biochemical Journal	http://www.portlandpress.co.uk/bj/default.htm	full journal

Journals *(continued)*

Blood and Bone Marrow Transplant newsletter	http://www.bmtnews.org	full journal
Blood Cells, Molecules, and Diseases	http://seconde.scripps.edu	full journal
Blood Weekly	http://www.newsfile.com	subscription
British Medical Journal	http://www.bmj.com	text
Bulletin of the History of Medicine	http://muse.jhu.edu/journals/ bulletin_of_the_history_of_medicine	subscription
Canadian Association of Radiologists Journal	http://www.cma.ca/journals	text
Canadian Bioethics Report	http://www.cma.ca/journals	full journal
The Canadian Journal of Physiology and Pharmacology	http://www.nrc.ca/cisti/journals/rjpp.html	subscription
Canadian J. of Plastic Surgery	http://www.pulsus.com/plastics/home.htm	full journal
The Canadian Journal of Respiratory Therapy	http://www.cma.ca/journals	text
Canadian J. of Rural Medicine	http://www.cma.ca/journals	text
Canadian Journal of Surgery	http://www.cma.ca/journals	text
Canadian Medical Assn. Journal	http://www.cma.ca/journals	text
Cancer	http://journals.wiley.com/cancer	subscription
Cancer Journal	http://www.infobiogen.fr/agora/journals/ cancer/homepage.htm	full journal
Cancer Online	http://www.wiley.com/OnLine.html	full journal
Cancer Weekly	http://www.newsfile.com	subscription
Caring	http://www.nahc.org/NAHC/CaringComm/caring.html	text
Cell	http://www.cellpress.com	abstracts
Cell Physiology	http://www.uth.tmc.edu/apstracts	abstracts
Clinical and Diagnostic Laboratory Immunology	http://www.asmusa.org/jnlsrc/journal.htm	abstracts
Clinical Diabetes	http://www.diabetes.org/Publications	abstracts
Clinical Microbiology Reviews	http://www.asmusa.org/jnlsrc/journal.htm	abstracts
Cosmetic Surgery Times	http://www.modernmedicine.com/cstimes	text
Clinical and Investigative Medicine	http://www.cma.ca/journals	text
Computers in Nursing	http://www.cini.com/cin/cin.htm	text
Dental Study Club OnLine J.	http://www.tambcd.edu/DentalCE/dsc	full journal
Dentistry On-line	http://www.cityscape.co.uk/journals/dent.htm	full journal
Dermatology Times	http://www.modernmedicine.com/derm	text
Diabetes	http://www.diabetes.org/Publications	abstracts
Diabetes Care	http://www.diabetes.org/Publications	abstracts
Diabetes Reviews	http://www.diabetes.org/Publications	abstracts
Diabetes Spectrum	http://www.diabetes.org/Publications	abstracts
Digestive Health and Nutrition	http://www.med.harvard.edu/publications/ Health_Publications/dhns.html	text
Digital Journal of Ophthamology	http://www.meei.harvard.edu/meei/DJOhome.html	text
Digital Urology Journal	http://www.duj.com	full journal
Disease Prevention News	http://www.tdh.state.tx.us/phpep/dpnhome.htm	full journal
Disease Weekly	http://www.newsfile.com	subscription

Journals *(continued)*

Educational Synopses in Anesthesiology and Critical Care Medicine	http://gasnet.med.yale.edu/esia	full journal
Emerging Infectious Diseases	http://www.cdc.gov/ncidod/EID/eid.htm	full journal
Endocrinology and Metabolism	http://www.uth.tmc.edu/apstracts	abstracts
Evidence-Based Medicine	http://www.acponline.org/journals/ebm/ebmmenu.htm	text
Experimental Biology Online	http://science.springer.de/ebo/ebo-main.htm	full journal
Family Practice On-line	http://www.CityScape.co.uk/journals/fam.htm	full journal
FDA News	http://www.fda.gov/opacom/hpnews.html	full journal
Fertility Weekly	http://www.newsfile.com	subscription
Formulary	http://www.modernmedicine.com/formulary	text
Gastrointestinal and Liver Physiology	http://www.uth.tmc.edu/apstracts	abstracts
Gene Therapy Weekly	http://www.newsfile.com	subscription
Genome Research	http://www.cshl.org	text
General Practice On-line	http://www.cityscape.co.uk/journals/gp.htm	full journal
Geriatric Medicine	http://www.docnet.org.uk	text
Geriatrics	http://www.modernmedicine.com/geri	abstracts
Good Health Magazine	http://www.goodhealth.com	text
Harvard Health Letter	http://www.med.harvard.edu/publications/ Health_Publications/hlns.html	text
Harvard Heart Letter	http://www.med.harvard.edu/publications/ Health_Publications/hrtns.html	text
Health Data Management	http://hdm.fgray.com	text
Health Letter on the CDC	http://www.newsfile.com	subscription
Health Management Technology	http://www.healthmgttech.com/index.html	text
Health Psychology	http://www.apa.org/journals/hea.html	abstracts
Health Services Research	http://www.xnet.com/~hret/hsr.htm	abstracts
Health Watch	http://www.hcfa.gov/news/newsltr.htm	full journal
Heart and Circulatory Physiology	http://www.uth.tmc.edu/apstracts	abstracts
HeartWeb	http://www.heartweb.org	full journal
Hepatitis Weekly	http://www.newsfile.com	subscription
Human Genome News	http://www.ornl.gov/TechResources/ Human_Genome/publicat/publications.html	full journal
Hypertension, Dialysis, and Clinical Nephrology	http://www.medtext.com/hdcn.shtml	abstracts
Immunity	http://www.cellpress.com	abstracts
Immunotherapy Weekly	http://www.newsfile.com	subscription
Infection and Immunity	http://www.asmusa.org/jnlsrc/journal.htm	abstracts
Infectious Diseases in Children	http://www.slackinc.com/child/idc/idchome.htm	text
Infectious Disease News	http://www.slackinc.com/general/idn/idnhome.htm	text
International Journal of Systematic Bacteriology	http://www.asmusa.org/jnlsrc/journal.htm	abstracts
Internet J. of Health Promotion	http://www.monash.edu.au/health/IJHP	full journal
Internet Journal of Ophthalmology	http://phobos.unich.it:80/injo	full journal
International Journal of Systematic Bacteriology	http://www.asmusa.org/jnlsrc/journal.htm	abstracts
Inter Nurse	http://www.kencomp.com/internurse	full journal

Journals *(continued)*

JAMA	http://www.ama-assn.org	text
Journal of AIDS/HIV	http://www.ccspublishing.com	full journal
Journal of the American College of Cardiology	http://www-east.elsevier.com/jac/jac_mnth.htm	text
Journal of Animal Science	http://www.asas.org	membership
Journal of Bacteriology	http://www.asmusa.org/jnlsrc/journal.htm	abstracts
Journal of Cell Science	http://www.CityScape.co.uk/users/ag64/jcsindex.htm	abstracts
Journal of Biological Chemistry	http://www-jbc.stanford.edu	subscription
J. of Clinical Microbiology	http://www.asmusa.org/jnlsrc/journal.htm	abstracts
Journal of Clinical Monitoring	gopher://gasnet.med.yale.edu	abstracts
Journal of Clinical Oncology	http://www.jcojournal.org/toc.html	abstracts
Journal Club on the Web	http://www.journalclub.org	abstracts
J. of Emergency Medicine Online	http://www.ccspublishing.com	full journal
Journal of Experimental Medicine	http://www.jem.org	abstracts
J. of Family Medicine Online	http://www.ccspublishing.com	full journal
The Journal of Family Practice	http://jfp.msu.edu	text
J. of Family Practice Journal Club	http://jfp.msu.edu/jclub/jclub.htm	text
Journal of Image Guided Surgery	http://www.igs.wiley.com	full journal
Journal of Immunology	http://journals.at-home.com	abstracts
J. of Informatics in Primary Care	http://www.ncl.ac.uk:80/~nphcare/PHCSG/Journal	text
Journal of Molecular Biology	http://www.hbuk.co.uk/jmb	subscription
J. of the National Cancer Institute	http://wwwicic.nci.nih.gov/jnci/jnci_issues.html	abstracts
Journal of Neonatal Nursing	http://www.bizjet.com/jnn	text
Journal of Neuroscience	http://www.jneurosci.org	abstracts
Journal of Neuroscience Nursing	http://www.prairienet.org/aann/jrnlabst.html	abstracts
J. of Neurosurgical Anesthesiology	gopher://gasnet.med.yale.edu	abstracts
Journal of Nursing Informatics	http://milkman.cac.psu.edu/~dxm12/OJNI.html	full journal
Journal of Nursing Jocularity	http://www.jocularity.com	text
Journal of Nursing Management	http://www.blacksci.co.uk/products/journals/jnm.htm	subscription
Journal of Nutrition	http://nutrition.org	abstracts
Journal of Obstetrics and Gynecology Online	http://www.ccspublishing.com	full journal
J. of Pediatric Medicine Online	http://www.ccspublishing.com	full journal
Journal of Physiology	http://physiology.cup.cam.ac.uk/index.html	abstracts
Journal of Primary Care On-Line	http://www.ccspublishing.com	full journal
Journal of Psychiatry Online	http://www.ccspublishing.com	full journal
Journal of Surgery Online	http://www.ccspublishing.com	full journal
The Journal of Urology	http://www.wwilkins.com/urology	abstracts
J. of Veterinary Med. Education	http://scholar.lib.vt.edu/ejournals/JVME/V21-1/tofc.html	full journal
Journal of Virology	http://www.asmusa.org/jnlsrc/journal.htm	abstracts
The Lancet	http://www.thelancet.com	abstracts
Lung Cellular and Molecular Physiology	http://www.uth.tmc.edu/apstracts	abstracts
Malaria and Tropical Disease Weekly	http://www.newsfile.com	subscription
Managed Healthcare	http://www.modernmedicine.com/mhc	text
Mayo Clinic Health O@sis	http://healthnet.ivi.com/ivi/mayo/common/htm/newsstnd.htm	full journal

Journals *(continued)*

MD Anderson Oncolog	http://www.mdacc.tmc.edu/~oncolog	full journal
Medical Journal of Australia	http://www.library.usyd.edu.au/MJA	text
The Medical Reporter	http://www.dash.com/netro/nwx/tmr/tmr.html	full journal
Medicine On-line	http://www.cityscape.co.uk/journals/med.htm	abstracts
Men's Health Watch	http://www.med.harvard.edu/publications/ Health_Publications/mnsns.html	text
Mental Health Letter	http://www.med.harvard.edu/publications/ Health_Publications/mntlns.html	text
Microbiology and Molecular Biology Reviews	http://www.asmusa.org/jnlsrc/journal.htm	abstracts
Modern Medicine	http://www.modernmedicine.com/modern	text
Molecular and Cellular Biology	http://www.asmusa.org/jnlsrc/journal.htm	abstracts
Morbidity and Mortality Weekly Report	http://www.cdc.gov/epo/mmwr/mmwr.html	full journal
Nature Medicine	http://medicine.nature.com/content	abstracts
Neuron	http://www.cellpress.com	abstracts
Neurosurgery	http://www.wwilkins.com/neurosurgery	text
NIH Clinical Alerts	gopher://gopher.nlm.nih.gov:70/11/alerts	full journal
Nutrition Action Health Letter	http://www.cspinet.org/nah	text
New England J. of Medicine	http://www.nejm.org	text
Nursing Review	http://nursing.camrev.com.au	abstracts
NurseWeek	http://www.nurseweek.com	full journal
Nursing Standard Online	http://www.nursing-standard.co.uk	text
Ocular Surgery News	http://www.slackinc.com/eye/osn/osnhome.htm	text
Online Journal of Cardiology	http://www.hrt.org	full journal
Online J. of Issues in Nursing	http://www.nursingworld.org/ojin	full journal
Online Journal of Knowledge Synthesis in Nursing	http://www.oclc.org/oclc/forms/ojksn.htm	subscription
Online J. of Nursing Informatics	http://milkman.cac.psu.edu/~dxm12/OJNI.html	full journal
Online J. of Veterinary Research	http://www.powerup.com.au/~jvet/jvet196a.htm	full journal
Ophthamology Times	http://www.modernmedicine.com/ot	text
Orthopedics Today	http://www.slackinc.com/bone/ortoday/othome.htm	text
Osler Medical Journal	http://omj.med.jhu.edu	full journal
Pediatric Pharmacotherapy	http://galen.med.virginia.edu/~smb4v/pedpharm/ pedpharm.html	full journal
Pediatric Surgery Today	http://home.coqui.net/titolugo	text
Pediatrics	http://www.pediatrics.org	text
Pharmacy Case Review	http://pharmacy.isu.edu:80/pcr/pcr.html	abstracts
Physicians Practice Digest	http://www.ppdnet.com	text
Physician Recruitment	http://www.ama-assn.org	text
Proceedings of the National Academy of Sciences	http://www.pnas.org	subscription, abstracts
Psychiatric Times	http://www.mhsource.com/psychiatrictimes.html	full journal
Psychiatry On-line	http://www.cityscape.co.uk/journals/psych.htm	abstracts
Regulatory, Integrative and Comparative Physiology	http://www.uth.tmc.edu/apstracts	abstracts
Renal Physiology	http://www.uth.tmc.edu/apstracts	abstracts
Science	http://www.sciencemag.org	subscription

Journals *(continued)*

Scientific American	http://www.scientificamerican.com	text
Sex Weekly	http://www.newsfile.com	subscription
St. Francis Journal of Medicine	http://www.sfhs.edu/journal	full journal
Stanford Healthlink	http://healthlink.stanford.edu/healthlink	text
Stanford Medicine	http://www-med.stanford.edu/MedCenter/communications/Stanmed	full journal
Today's Internist	http://www.asim.org	full journal
Tuberculosis Weekly	http://www.newsfile.com	subscription
Urology Times	http://www.modernmedicine.com/ut	text
Vaccine Weekly	http://www.newsfile.com	subscription
Vet Online	http://www.priory.co.uk/journals/vet.htm	full journal
Virtual J.of Clinical Orthodontics	http://vjco.it	full journal
Weekly Epidemiological Record	http://www.who.ch/wer/wer_home.htm	full journal
Women's Health Watch	http://www.med.harvard.edu/publications/Health_Publications/whns.html	text
Women's Health Weekly	http://www.newsfile.com	subscription

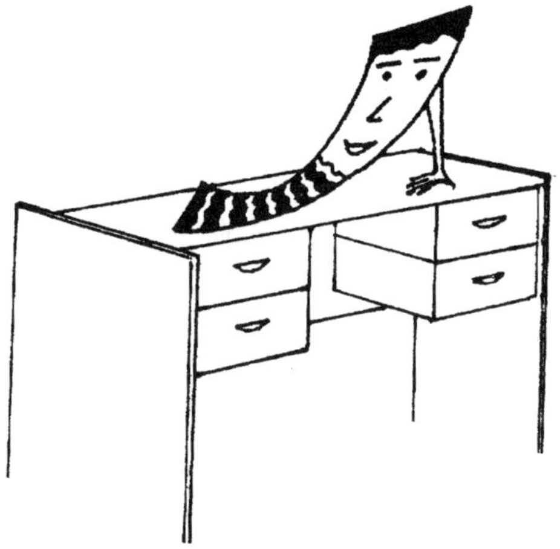

Chapter 12: Medical Sites

Of all the questions the one he asks most insistently is about man. How does he walk? How does the heart pump blood? What happens when he yawns and sneezes?

Sir Kenneth Clark, on Leonardo da Vinci

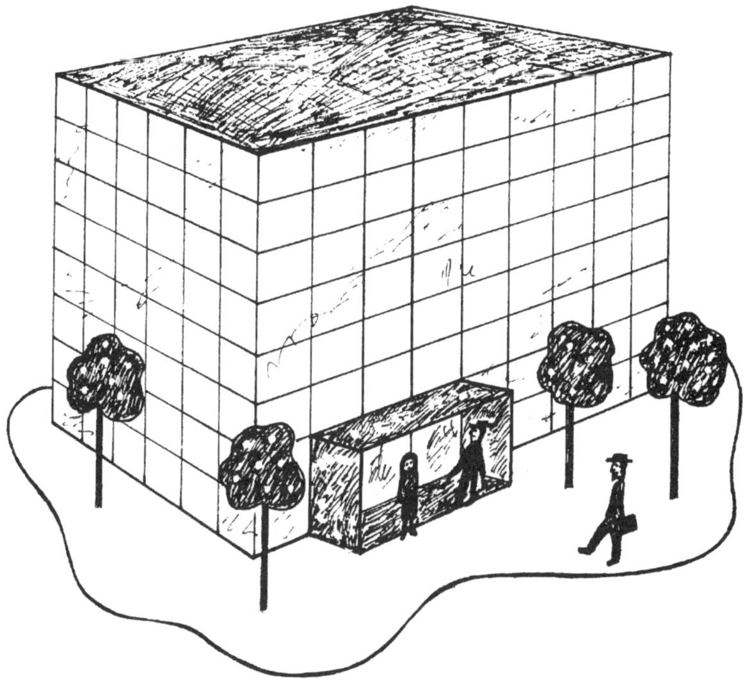

This chapter lists Web sites related to a specific medical specialty or topic. Keep in mind that there are more than 10,000 medical sites. This list is just a starting point.

With the number of sites so large and the Internet growing so fast, it is impractical to list smaller Web sites. The criteria for inclusion in this directory are:

- the site is a leader in its field
- the site contains a well-organized, easy to use set of links
- the site contains significant resources

Sometimes the best site is an area in one of the established directories (MedWeb, MedMark, Hardin, HealthAtoZ, Achoo, Galaxy). In any case they are always a reliable starting point.

Commercial "One-Stop" Medical Sites

The Internet now includes a number of commercial medical sites. Most of these are free, supported by advertising banners, but registration is often required. A few are open only to physicians, or available only by subscription. Commercial sites may be primarily for consumers (HealthAnswers), professionals (MedConnect), or both (HealthGate).

A commercial site will often advertise itself as a one-stop place to get all your medical information on the Internet, in the same way that America Online or Compuserve once tried to be all-inclusive info-malls for general topics. But in my opinion that strategy is short-sighted on the Internet, where so many important resources are available from so many different sites. If a person doesn't want to deal with different Web sites, or hasn't learned the basics of searching, then a single, limited commercial site may be useful. But commercial sites cannot yet match the much more extensive information from government (CDC, NIH) educational institutions (MedWeb, Virtual Hospital) and professional organizations (AMA).

In other words, if you feel more comfortable with a limited set of choices, or don't want to go looking for medical information, a commercial site might be just the thing. Remember that in a year or two the situation may change, and one of these sites could grow into a predominant medical site, just as the online bookstore Amazon.com (http://www.amazon.com) has done.

Commercial Sites

Avicenna	http://www.avicenna.com	Professionals. Registration. Medline.
HealthGate	http://www.healthgate.com	Public & professionals. Medline, other databases, patient education, texts, document delivery.
MedConnect	http://www.medconnect.com	Professionals. CME, rounds, jobs line, forums.
Medscape	http://www.medscape.com	Public and professionals. Medline, journal articles, patient education.
MedSource	http://www.medsource.com	Professionals. For executives, healthcare leaders.
NetMedicine	http://www.netmedicine.com	Professionals. Medline, rounds, patient education, photo rounds.
Physician's Guide to the Internet	http://www.webcom.com/pgi	Professionals. Mostly links to other sites.
Physicians' Online	http://www.po.com	Professionals. CME, Medline. Proprietary software. Version for non-MD professionals.
Physicians' Home Page	http://php.silverplatter.com/physicians	Professionals. CME. Subscription. Medline, links, drugs.

Medical Sites

(Links available at http://NewWindPub.com/workbook)

AIDS

AIDS Resource List	http://www.teleport.com/~celinec/aids.shtml
AIDS Resource Sampler	http://www.nnlm.nlm.nih.gov/pnr/etc/aidspath.html
CDC Ntl. AIDS Clearinghouse	gopher://cdcnac.aspensys.com
MedWeb	http://www.gen.emory.edu/MEDWEB/keyword/AIDS_and_HIV.html
Ntl. Inst. of Allergy/Infectious Dis.	gopher://odie.niaid.nih.gov:70/11/aids

ALTERNATIVE MEDICINE

HealthAtoZ	http://www.healthatoz.com/categories/AM.htm
Holistic Internet Resources	http://www.hir.com
MedWeb	http://www.gen.emory.edu/MEDWEB/keyword/ alternative_medicine.html

ANATOMY

Human Anatomy Resources	http://www.sunshine.net/folkstone/anatomist/anatomy
MedWeb	http://www.gen.emory.edu/MEDWEB/keyword/ anatomy_and_embryology.html

ANESTHESIOLOGY

GASNet	http://gasnet.med.yale.edu
MedMark	http://medmark.bit.co.kr/ane2.html

ASSOCIATIONS

American Medical Assn.	http://www.ama-assn.org/med_link/nation.htm
MedWeb	http://www.gen.emory.edu/medweb/medweb.societies.html

BIOETHICS

MedWeb	http://www.gen.emory.edu/MEDWEB/keyword/bioethics.html
UB Ctr. for Clinical Ethics	http://wings.buffalo.edu/faculty/research/bioethics

BIOSTATISTICS

Biostatistics	http://www.biostat.washington.edu/Xvlib
Links to Biometry	http://WWW.AMS.Med.Uni-Goettingen.DE/~rhilger/Biometry.html

CARDIOLOGY

American Heart Association	http://www.amhrt.org
Cardiology Compass	http://osler.wustl.edu/~murphy/cardiology/compass.html
MedMark	http://medmark.bit.co.kr/cardiol.html

CONFERENCES

Doctor's Guide (medical)	http://www.pslgroup.com/MEDCONF.HTM
Doctor's Guide (nursing)	http://www.pslgroup.com/dg/Nursing.htm
MedWeb	http://www.gen.emory.edu/medweb/medweb.conferences.html

DENTISTRY

Am. Acad. of Pediatric Dentistry	http://www.aapd.org
American Dental Assn.	http://www.ada.org
Dental-Related Internet List	http://www.citizen.infi.net/~dmtrop/dental/dental3.html
Dental-Related Internet Resources	http://www.dental-resources.com

DERMATOLOGY

Internet Dermatology Society	http://www.telemedicine.org/ids.htm
U. of Iowa Dept. of Dermatology	http://tray.dermatology.uiowa.edu

DISABILITY

Disabled Peoples International	http://www.escape.ca/~dpi
disABILITY Information	http://www.eskimo.com/~jlubin/disabled.html

DISEASES

CliniWeb	http://www.ohsu.edu/cliniweb/disease.html
HealthAtoZ	http://www.healthatoz.com/categories/DC.htm
Karolinska Institute	http://www.mic.ki.se/Diseases
MedicineNet	http://www.medicinenet.com

EDUCATION

Apple Education Worldwide	http://hed.info.apple.com/med
Interactive Med Student Lounge	http://www.geocities.com/Heartland/1756/lounge.html
Medical Schools	http://www.aamc.org/meded/start.htm
Nursing	http://www.lib.umich.edu/hw/nursing.html
MedWeb	http://www.gen.emory.edu/medweb/medweb.ed.html

EMERGENCY MEDICINE

Emerg. Medicine and Prim. Care	http://www.embbs.com
MedWeb	http://www.gen.emory.edu/medweb/medweb.emergency.html
Safety Related Internet Resources	http://www.mrg.ab.ca/christie/safelist.htm
Web of Emergency Services	http://dumbo.isc.rit.edu/ems/index.html

EMPLOYMENT (see also table at the end of Chapter 18)

Achoo	http://www.achoo.com/achoo/business/companie/employme.htm
MedSearch	http://www.medsearch.com
MedWeb	http://www.gen.emory.edu/medweb/medweb.jobs.html

ENDOCRINOLOGY

Diabetic Data Centre	http://www.demon.co.uk/diabetic
Diabetes Monitor	http://www.mdcc.com
MedWeb	http://www.gen.emory.edu/medweb/medweb.endocrinology.html
NIDDK	http://www.niddk.nih.gov

FAMILY MEDICINE

Family & Int. Med., Prim. Care	http://www.nmmc.com/libweb/medstaff/famlymed.htm
Family Medicine Links	http://jfp.msu.edu/fammed.htm
MedWeb	http://www.gen.emory.edu/MEDWEB/keyword/family_medicine.html
Primary Care Internet Resources	http://views.vcu.edu/views/fap/volc-r.html

FORENSICS

Zeno's Forensic Page	http://www.bart.nl:80/~geradts/forensic.html

GASTROENTEROLOGY

American Gastroenterology Assn.	http://www.gastro.org
Gastroenterology Web	http://cpmcnet.columbia.edu/dept/gi
MedMark	http://medmark.bit.co.kr/gastro.html
MedWeb	http://www.gen.emory.edu/medweb/medweb.gastroenterology.html

GENETICS

Human Genome Project	http://www.ornl.gov/TechResources/Human_Genome
Molecular Genetics Jump Station	http://www.ifrn.bbsrc.ac.uk/gm/lab/docs/genetics.html
Resources for Molecular Biology	http://www.medcor.mcgill.ca/EXPMED/DOCS/resource.html

GERIATRICS

Administration on Aging	http://www.aoa.dhhs.gov
Eldercare Web	http://www.elderweb.com
Seniors Computer Info Project	http://www.mbnet.mb.ca/crm

GOVERNMENT

Achoo	http://www.achoo.com/achoo/practice/governme/index.htm
Ag. for Health Care Policy & Res.	http://www.ahcpr.gov
Centers for Disease Control	http://www.cdc.gov
Dept. of Health and Human Svcs.	http://www.os.dhhs.gov
FedWorld	http://www.fedworld.gov
Food and Drug Administration	http://www.fda.gov
Health Care Financing Admin.	http://www.hcfa.gov
Health Care Reform	http://www.gen.emory.edu/medweb/medweb.healthreform.html
Indian Health Service	http://www.tucson.ihs.gov
National Institutes of Health	http://www.nih.gov
Occup. Safety and Health Admin.	http://www.osha.gov
Social Security Administration	http://www.ssa.gov
United Nations	http://www.un.org
Veterans Administration	http://www.va.gov
World Health Administration	http://www.who.ch

GRANTS and RESEARCH

MedWeb	http://www.gen.emory.edu/medweb/medweb.grants.html
Resources for Inst. Research	http://apollo.gmu.edu/~jmilam/air95.html

HISTORY OF MEDICINE

Australian Science Archives Proj.	http://www.asap.unimelb.edu.au

HOSPICE

Death, Dying and Grief Resources	http://www.cyberspy.com/~webster/death.html
Hospice Hands	http://hospice-cares.com

HOSPITALS

Health on the Net	http://www.hon.ch
HospitalWeb	http://neuro-www.mgh.harvard.edu/hospitalweb.nclk
MedAccess	http://www.medaccess.com

IMMUNOLOGY

MedWeb	http://www.gen.emory.edu/medweb/medweb.immunology.html
MedMark	http://medmark.bit.co.kr/immunol.html
Ntl. Inst. of Allergy and Inf. Dis.	http://www.niaid.nih.gov
Ntl. Jewish Center for Immun.	http://www.njc.org

INFECTIOUS DISEASE

Centers for Disease Control	http://www.cdc.gov
Communicable Disease Surveillance Center	http://www.open.gov.uk/cdsc

INFORMATICS

Am. Medical Informatics Assn.	http://www.amia.org
Medical Informatics at Stanford	http://www-camis.stanford.edu
MedWeb	http://www.gen.emory.edu/medweb/medweb.informatics.html

JOURNALS (see also Chapter 11)

American Medical Association	http://www.ama-assn.org
Ecola Directories	http://www.ecola.com/news/magazine/health
Elec. Journals in Health Sciences	http://www.hslib.washington.edu/journals
Electronic Newsstand	http://www.enews.com/monster/health
Journals in Biosciences	http://golgi.harvard.edu/journals.html
MedWeb	http://www.gen.emory.edu/MEDWEB/alphakey/electronic_publications.html
Medworld	http://www.med.stanford.edu/medworld/research_journals.html

LIBRARIES

Library of Congress links	http://lcweb.loc.gov/z3950
MedWeb	http://www.gen.emory.edu/medweb/medweb.medlibs.html

MICROBIOLOGY

All the Virology on the WWW	http://www.tulane.edu/~dmsander/garryfavweb.html
LSU World of Medical Sciences	http://www.lsumc.edu/campus/micr/www.htm

NEPHROLOGY

Kidney and Urologic Diseases	http://www.hsls.pitt.edu/subjects/kidney.html
Nephron Information Center	http://www.nephron.com
Renal Net	http://ns.gamewood.net/renalnet.html

NEUROLOGY

Neurosciences on the Internet	http://www.lm.com/~nab
Neurosciences at the UW	http://weber.u.washington.edu/~wcalvin/neuro-uw.html
Virtual Library; Neuroscience	http://neuro.med.cornell.edu/VL

NEUROSURGERY

Neurosurgical WWW Sites	http://www.abdn.ac.uk/~u01ng/anand.htm
Am. Assn. of Neuro Surgeons	http://www.aans.org

NURSING

Am. Journal of Nursing	http://www.ajn.org
Am. Nurses Association	http://www.nursingworld.org
Kentucky Coal. of Nurse Pract.	http://www.achiever.com/freehmpg/kynurses
MedWeb	http://www.gen.emory.edu/medweb/medweb.nursing.html
Nightingale	http://nightingale.con.utk.edu
Nursing & Health Care Resources on the Net	http://www.shef.ac.uk/~nhcon
Nursing Net	http://www.nursingnet.org
U. of Michigan	http://www.lib.umich.edu/hw/nursing.html

NUTRITION

Food and Nutrition Info Center	http://www.nal.usda.gov/fnic
The Food Resource	http://www.orst.edu/food-resource/food.html
MedWeb	http://www.gen.emory.edu/medweb/medweb.nutrition.html

OBSTETRICS

MedWeb	http://www.gen.emory.edu/medweb/medweb.gynecology.html
MedWeb	http://www.gen.emory.edu/medweb/medweb.reproductive.html
Ob/Gyn Net	http://www.obgyn.net
Reproduction and Women's Health	http://www.med.upenn.edu/~crrwh/ScientificSites.html

OCCUPATIONAL HEALTH

OSHWeb	http://turva.me.tut.fi/~oshweb
Safety Links Directory	http://www.pro-am.com/safelink.htm

ONCOLOGY

CancerNet	http://wwwicic.nci.nih.gov
Cancer News on the Net	http://www.cancernews.com/quickload.htm
Hardin	http://www.arcade.uiowa.edu/hardin-www/md-oncol.html
Oncolink	http://cancer.med.upenn.edu

OPHTHAMOLOGY

Am. Assn. for Pediatric Ophthalmology and Strabismus	http://med-aapos.bu.edu
Ophthamology Sites on the Web	http://www.web-xpress.com/athens/webopht.html
Vision Science	http://vision.arc.nasa.gov/VisionScience

ORTHOPEDICS

Orthopaedic Links Page	http://www.virtualkamloops.com/cloughs/orthlink.html
U. of D. Ortho & Trauma Surgery	http://www.dundee.ac.uk/orthopaedics

OTOLARYNGOLOGY

Assn. for Research in Otol.	http://www.aro.org
Mt. Sinai Dept. of Otol.	http://www.mssm.edu/ent

PATHOLOGY

HealthWeb Pathology	http://www.biomed.lib.umn.edu/healthweb/labmedpathology.html
Univ. of Michigan	http://www.pds.med.umich.edu/users/amp/path_resources.html

PEDIATRICS

Am. Acad. of Pediatrics	http://www.aap.org
Neonatology on the Web	http://www.csmc.edu/neonatology/default.html
Univ. of Alabama PEDINFO	http://www.uab.edu/pedinfo

PHARMACOLOGY

Gold Multimedia Database	http://www.cponline.gsm.com
HealthWeb	http://omni.cc.purdue.edu/~wrunning/hw
PDRNet	http://www.pdrnet.com
PharmInfo	http://pharminfo.com
RxList	http://www.rxlist.com
RxMed	http://www.rxmed.com
Virtual Library; Pharmacy	http://www.cpb.uokhsc.edu/pharmacy/pharmint.html

PHYSICAL MEDICINE & REHABILITATION

Marquette U. PT Links	http://www.mu.edu/dept/pt/otherlinks.html
MedWeb	http://www.gen.emory.edu/medweb/medweb.rehab.html
Physical Therapy Central	http://www.ptcentral.com
Virtual Hospital	http://indy.radiology.uiowa.edu

PHYSICIAN ASSISTANTS

Am. Acad. of Physician Assts.	http://www.aapa.org
Medweb	http://www.gen.emory.edu/medweb/medweb.pa.html
PA Page	http://www.papage.com/papage

PHYSICS, CHEMISTRY, BIOLOGY

BiotTechNet Biology Resources	http://www.biotechniques.com/biosrc.html
MedWeb	http://www.gen.emory.edu/MEDWEB/keyword/biophysics.html

PHYSIOLOGY

Virtual Lib; Phys. & Biophysics	http://physiology.med.cornell.edu/WWWVL/PhysioWeb.html

PODIATRY

Podiatry Online	http://207.158.247.38/footman/
Am. Podiatric Medical Assn	http://www.apma.org

PREVENTIVE MEDICINE

Health Promotion on the Internet	http://www.monash.edu.au/health

PRODUCTS AND SERVICES

Achoo	http://www.achoo.com/achoo/business/medical
Medicom	http://www.medicom.com

PSYCHIATRY

FreudNet	http://plaza.interport.net/nypsan/network.html
Guide to Psychotherapy	http://www.shef.ac.uk/~psysc/psychotherapy
Internet Mental Health Resources	http://www.med.nyu.edu/Psych/src.psych.html
Inst. of Psychiatry Library	http://www.iop.bpmf.ac.uk/home/depts/library/ment.htm
Mental Health Net	http://www.cmhc.com

PUBLIC HEALTH

Hardin	http://www.arcade.uiowa.edu/hardin-www/md-publ.html
Health Svcs & Public Health Sites	http://weber.u.washington.edu/~larsson/hsic94/resource/hsr-ph.html
MedWeb	http://www.gen.emory.edu/medweb/medweb.ph.html
Public Health Resources on the Internet	http://www.lib.berkeley.edu/PUBL/internet.html

PULMONARY

Respiratory Hot Links	http://www.xmission.com/~gastown/herpmed/respi.htm
MedWeb	http://www.gen.emory.edu/medweb/medweb.respmed.html

RADIOLOGY

Am. College of Radiology	http://www.acr.org
Medical Imaging Resources	http://pubweb.acns.nwu.edu/~dbk675/netsites.html
Medical Imaging Resources	http://agora.leeds.ac.uk/comir/resources/links.html
Radiological Soc. of N. Am	http://www.rsna.org

RHEUMATOLOGY

HealthWeb	http://www.medlib.iupui.edu/hw/rheuma/home.html
MedWeb	http://www.gen.emory.edu/MEDWEB/keyword/rheumatology.html

SPORTS MEDICINE

Biomechanics World Wide	http://dragon.acadiau.ca/~pbaudin/biomch.html
MedWeb	http://www.gen.emory.edu/medweb/medweb.sportsmed.html

SUBSTANCE ABUSE

Drug and Alcohol Treatment Net	http://www.datnet.com
Join Together Online	http://www.jointogether.org
Prevention Online	http://www.health.org
Web of Addictions	http://www.well.com/user/woa

SURGERY

Karolinska	http://www.mic.ki.se/Diseases/e4.html
MedMark	http://medmark.bit.co.kr/general.html
MedWeb	http://www.gen.emory.edu/medweb/medweb.surgery.html
Trauma.org	http://www.trauma.org

TELEMEDICINE

Telemedicine Links	http://www.jma.com.au/telelink.htm
Telemedicine Resources	http://icsl.ee.washington.edu/~cabralje/tmresources.html

TESTS AND PROCEDURES

HealthAnswers	http://www.healthanswers.com
Health Gate	http://www.healthgate.com

TEXTBOOKS AND REFERENCE

Family Practice Handbook	http://vh.radiology.uiowa.edu/Providers/ClinRef/FPHandbook/FPContents.html
Medical Dictionary	http://www.drschueler.com/glossary/glossary.htm
MedicineNet	http://www.medicinenet.com
Merck Manual	http://www.merck.com
Multilingual Glossary	http://allserv.rug.ac.be/~rvdstich/eugloss/welcome.html
Surgical Glossary	http://www.mtdesk.com/swg.shtml

TOXICOLOGY

MedWeb	http://www.gen.emory.edu/MEDWEB/keyword/toxicology.html
Toxicology Resource	http://www.pitt.edu/~martint

TRANSPLANTATION

CenterSpan	http://www.centerspan.org/
Transplant Desk Reference	http://www.asf.org/tdr.html
TransWeb	http://www.transweb.org

VETERINARY MEDICINE

HealthWeb Veterinary Medicine	http://www.lib.msu.edu/publ_ser/branches/ccl/lxb/vetmed.htm
MedWeb	http://www.gen.emory.edu/medweb/medweb.vet.html
Virginia-Maryland College Links	http://www.vetmed.vt.edu

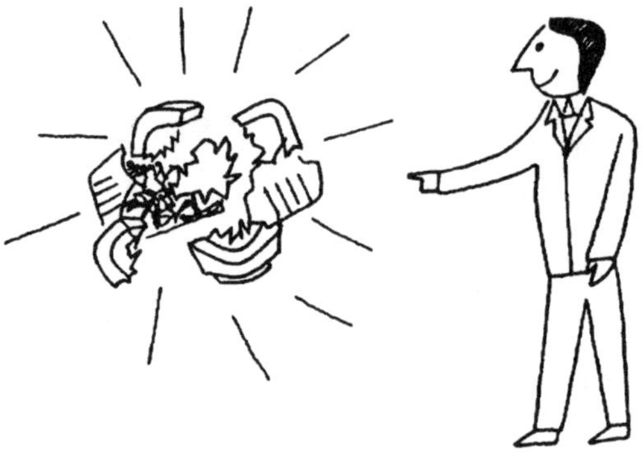

Part Three:
Professional Skills

Ethics, Law, Responsibility
Mailing Lists, Discussion Groups
Managing Time and Information
Troubleshooting
Creating Information
New Career Choices

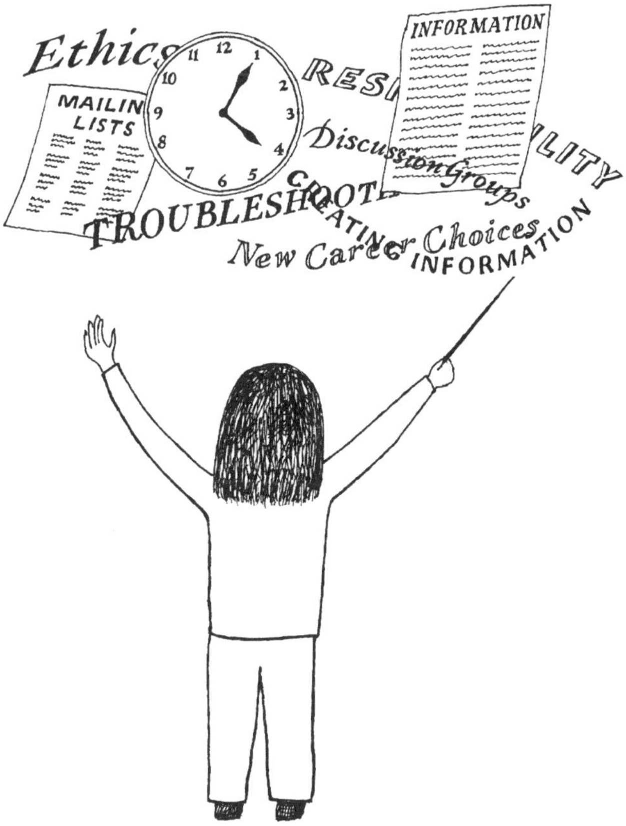

After finishing Part Three, you will be able to:

- *Subscribe to and participate in a mailing list*
- *Read and post messages to a newsgroup*
- *Troubleshoot basic computer and Internet problems*

Chapter 13: Ethics, Law, Responsibility

Words are also actions, and actions are a kind of words.

Ralph Waldo Emerson

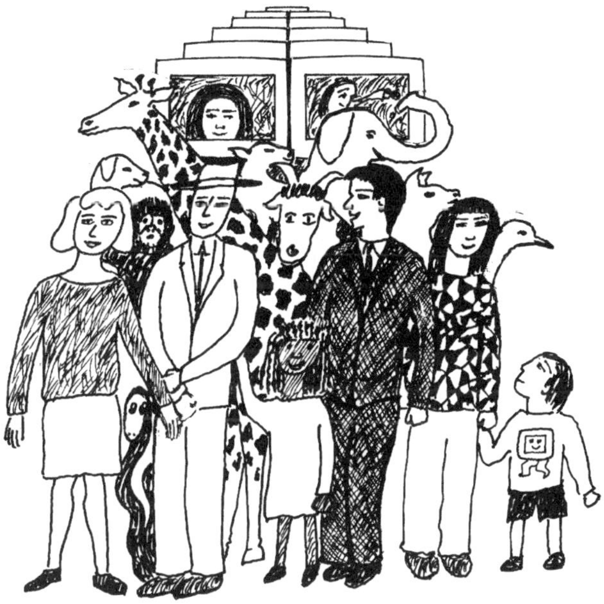

IN THIS CHAPTER

- censorship
- confidentiality
- copyright
- defamatory
- disclosure
- encryption
- ethics
- fair use
- informed consent
- liability
- libel
- license limitation
- negligence
- privacy
- professional relationships
- professional responsibility
- rights
- scope of practice
- slander

Introduction

Technology and Healthcare

New kinds of communication enter our lives every few years; many of them are used heavily in healthcare. Look at the hospital where I work. We have an in-house television channel, and we produce a weekly program for a public station. Several Web servers supply information for the Internet. Bedside nurses have pagers. Respiratory technicians have portable computers. Everybody in administration has a voice mailbox.

Almost every modern office, clinic and hospital has a fax machine, which is often used to transmit clinical information such as chart summaries. Email is commonplace in large hospitals, and increasingly used for collaborative projects. Telemedicine is being developed in many centers. These changes affect all of us, and we need to understand the basic ethical and legal principles that apply to communication.

The Mark of a Professional

Expertise with communication is <u>the</u> mark of a professional, much more so than any other skill. Learning a body of knowledge is half your education; learning to

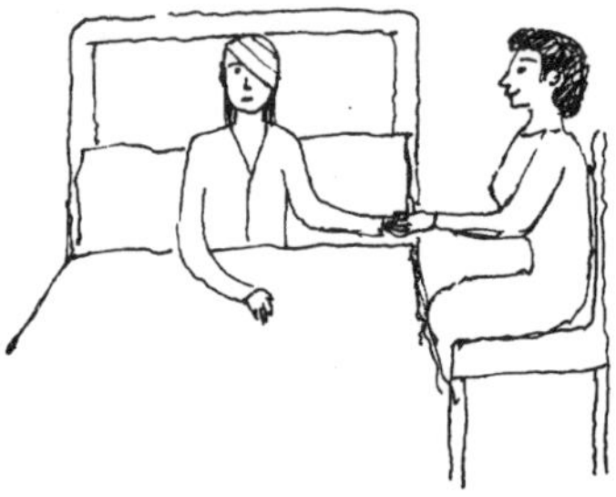

teach is the other half. "We have to close the distance between the push-button order and the human act. We have to touch people." (Jacob Bronowski)

As a professional in the modern world you will be working with voice mail, email, Web forums, teleconferencing, and other methods that have not even been created yet. As a professional you will be expected to uphold certain standards of conduct, whether they are explicit or implicit.

Basic Principles

Slander and Libel

> Every person is legally responsible for what he says and writes.

The first amendment to the Constitution of the United States guarantees the right to free speech, but every person is responsible for what he says and writes. If you make certain kinds of statements in speech or writing you can be sued in a court of law.

A defamatory statement is one that subjects a person, group, or institution to hatred, contempt or ridicule, or one that results in injury to a business or work reputation. One example is accusing a person of illegal activity. You might write a letter to the paper stating that your next door neighbor is a thief. If you make a written statement that is defamatory, you can be sued for libel; if you make a spoken statement that is defamatory, you can be sued for slander. Anytime you criticize another, you are skating on thin ice. "Angry words hurt, and the hurt rebounds." (*Dhammapada*, trans. Thomas Byron)

A slightly different standard applies to persons who are public figures, because it is expected that there will be public discussion about them. Politicians, news reporters, professional athletes, television and movie actors are public figures. In some cases it is unclear whether a person is a public figure or not, and this must be decided in court.

For a statement about a public figure to be defamatory, it must be proved that the statement was made with actual malice, meaning that the person who made it knew that it was false, or had a reckless disregard for the truth or falsity of the statement.

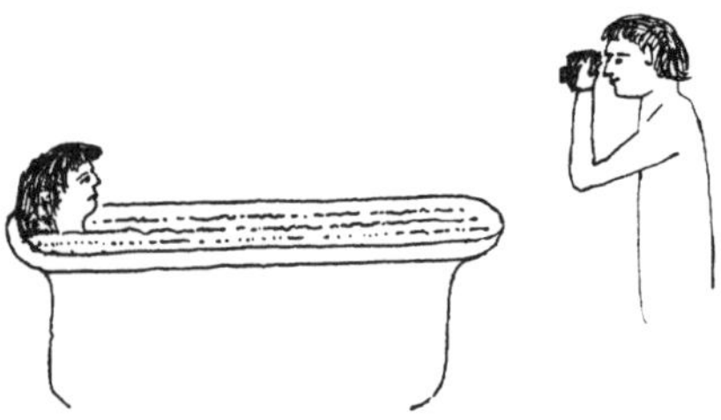

Privacy

Something that is private is kept out of public view. The law recognizes that certain aspects of a person's life are private and that if you violate a person's privacy you can be held liable in a court of law. The exact interpretation of privacy, however, varies from state to state.

It is not against the law to take pictures of a person while he is in a public place, such as the park. But if you take pictures in a person's home, you have entered his "private domain" and have intruded upon his seclusion. The pictures need not be published for you to be held liable.

Another way that privacy can be violated is by public disclosure of private facts. A private fact is one that a person would reasonably wish to keep to oneself, such as a history of psychiatric illness. Again, public figures are held to a different standard. If a disclosure of a fact is truthful and bears some relationship to a public role, it may not be deemed an invasion of privacy.

On the Internet there are many issues related to privacy. Web browsers can transmit information about you, including your operating system, your service provider, and which Web site you visited last. With cookies (see Chapter 4), a Web site can save information on your own computer. Email can be intercepted.

There are various technical ways to safeguard privacy, such as encryption, but these are not foolproof. In general, you shouldn't assume that any message or file that you send over the Internet will be kept private.

Encryption is not foolproof.

The same is true of computer files. People have discovered, to their dismay, that files which they thought were deleted can be restored. If you have sensitive information, don't store it on a computer at work which others can access, or which might be taken for repair at any time. This might apply to an electronic addressbook kept at work as well.

Health Professionals

Standard of Care

A different standard applies to healthcare providers than to the public at large regarding actions and words in relation to a patient. When you take care of a person, your interaction now falls into the category of professional relationship, and you must act, speak and write accordingly.

Healthcare providers are held to a professional standard.

A professional relationship exists as soon as you provide care to another person. *That care need not be in the place or time of your work.* If you give nursing care to a friend in her home, the same standards apply as if you were doing it in a clinic.

Teaching is one kind of care; remember that many healthcare providers do not perform hands-on physical care, but are still considered to be practicing medicine or nursing. In other words, *it is possible to set up a professional relationship through the spoken or written word.*

Teaching is a type of patient care.

Liability and Negligence

Each person is responsible for his actions and words. If actions or words cause harm, a person can be held liable in a court of law. As a professional you have an additional standard to uphold. You are expected to act as would another reasonable professional would who has your training, skills, and experience. If you fail to act in this way, you can be held negligent.

Informed Consent

Healthcare providers must obtain informed consent before performing any procedure or treatment on a person. Informed consent means that a person fully understands the treatment before agreeing that it be done. Consent is usually obtained in writing. Hospitals often require that patients sign a general consent for standard nursing procedures upon admission, and then individual consent for specific treatments.

Confidentiality

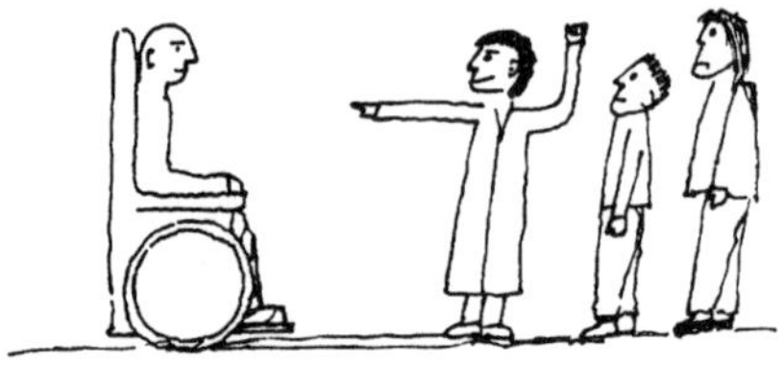

As a healthcare provider you are expected to keep your knowledge of a patient confidential. This applies to information you obtain by reading a chart, looking up results on a computer, talking to the patient, discussing the patient with another provider, and so on. You cannot discuss what you know about a patient with friends, family, or the public. If you are using email to correspond with another professional about a patient, consider using a pseudonym such as P or X12 or AA instead of the person's name. This may protect the patient's confidentiality if the message is inadvertently sent to the wrong place or forwarded to another.

Scope of Practice

Each state licenses healthcare providers and determines the scope of practice for a particular profession. Standards vary from state to state. A physician, physician's aide, licensed practical nurse, registered nurse, and nurse's aide may have different limitations on what can be done in the practice of their respective professions.

Copyright Issues

Copyright

An author's right to control the use of what is created.

When a person writes an article, creates a slide show, takes a photograph, or records a movie clip, she has created "intellectual property," and copyright laws protect that work from being used inappropriately by others. Copyright is the right to protect your work from being copied by others without your permission. The law which determines most details in this regard is the Copyright Revision Act of 1976. (Internationally, the Berne Convention and the Universal Copyright Convention are the most important. The United States and Canada have signed both of these.)

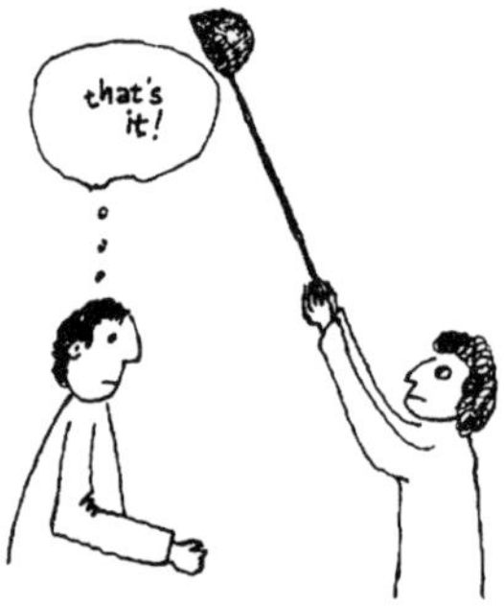

Stealing an idea

The moment that an article is "fixed in a tangible medium," such as printed on paper or saved to computer disk, it is protected by copyright. That copyright extends for the life of the author plus fifty years.

Copyright applies to the form or expression of a work, <u>not</u> to the ideas or concepts in it. An idea cannot be copyrighted; if I tell another nurse my idea for a great research project and she does the research first, she has not broken any laws. But if she copies a draft research paper and publishes it as her own, that is another matter.

Copyright includes five different rights: the right to reproduce a work, the right to produce a derivative work from it, the right to distribute copies for sale or lease, the right to perform it publicly, and the right to display it publicly. An author can sell or assign any of these rights to another person.

Work done as an employee is considered a work for hire, and the copyright belongs to the company, not the person who created the work. If you work for a university, there may be a special clause in your contract specifying the rights to any writing, research or development you do on the job.

What will happen to copyright as the tangible medium of paper is replaced by electronic bits? Nobody really knows. John Perry Barlow, founder of the Electronic Frontier Foundation (http://www.cff.org), one of the foremost organizations related to rights and privacy on the Internet, writes: "Digital technology is...erasing the legal jurisdictions of the physical world and replacing them with the unbounded and perhaps permanently lawless seas of cyberspace."

Fair Use

Every educator struggles with this dilemma: do I spend long hours researching and writing, or do I use the work that someone else has done? What if I copy an article to use in a class?

Copyright law allows for certain uses of copyrighted materials to be allowed as fair use. These include "purposes such as criticism, comment, news reporting, teaching (including multiple copies for classroom use), scholarship or research." But the law is ambiguous in this respect, and several factors are applied to any single case:

- What is the purpose of the use? Commercial or non-profit?
- How much of the original was used?
- What is the nature of the original work?
- Does the use affect the potential market or value of the work?

> ***Fair Use***
>
> Guidelines for the use of small portions of a copyrighted work without asking the author.

Technology and Humanity

Fear of the unknown often keeps us away from new technologies, but the ostrich approach is ultimately self-defeating. It's better to understand the essential issues, and then find a way to integrate these new tools into your life. If you wish to advance as a professional I guarantee you will need to know how to use computers, fax machines, email, voice mail, and the Internet.

Start at the Beginning

The first step for most professionals is to learn how to type. I recently met a director of a medical program who told me that when he realized how handicapped he was by not being able to type quickly, he took time off to learn. In today's world, not knowing how to type is equivalent to not knowing how to dial a telephone.

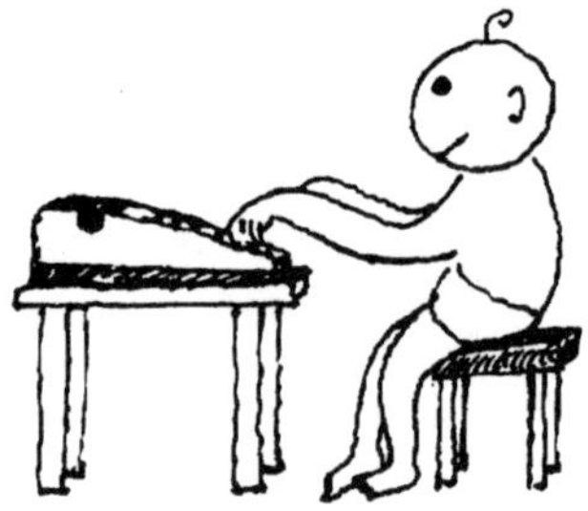

Toddler tip-tap

Ground Rules

In general, don't send any message that you wouldn't want published on the front page tomorrow—or sent to a worldwide newsgroup. When you send a message using electronic technology, that message can easily be stored and reproduced. Email is more public than most people imagine.

Don't say or write anything that is derogatory to another person or group. You may imagine that you are being witty, but such remarks can hurt your reputation, even if they are not illegal.

We are too familiar with language, most of us, to appreciate its complexity and nuances. We dash off an email message and press "Send" without thinking about how the other person will read it. Is the tone too intimate? Too brusque? Did I fall into a jargon that she won't understand? Have I used slang that might be offensive? Any misspelled words? Once you learn how you normally write, you can work to improve your writing with methods such as paraphrase, emphasis, metaphor, and anecdote. Every email message you send will then have the meaning and effect you want.

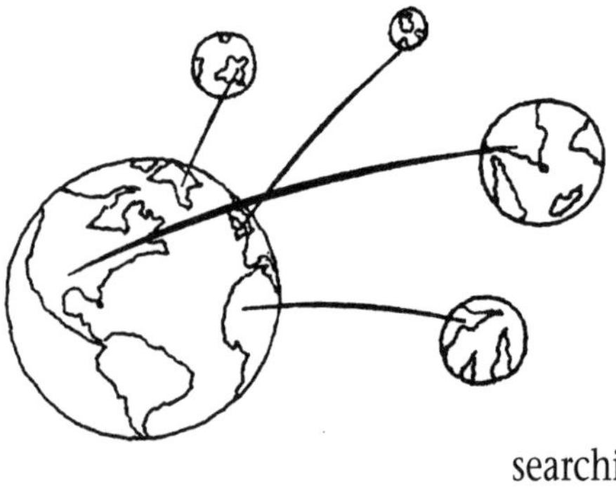

A Future World, One and Many

The email portion of Netscape Communicator includes the ability to send a message as a Web document, formatted so it can be placed on the Web immediately. This is a harbinger of the future, when different modes of communication (email, Web, pagers, voice mail) will increasingly be integrated. Messages will be sorted, archived in databases, accessible for searching by topic, convertible into other formats.

The development of all this will take time (if you are optimistic, a few months; pessimistic, a few decades) but expect it: communication technology will continue to move forward.

In the beginning the Internet was dominated by a spirit of cooperation, good will, and moral responsibility. Now that commerce is the fastest growing part of the Net, profit and advertising have eclipsed these more healthy and fundamental notions. Still, each of us is responsible for maintaining the highest standards possible.

EXERCISES

II. Problem-Solving

- Go to MedWeb (see table) and find the AMA Code of Medical Ethics, the Hippocratic Oath, and the Univ. of Pennsylvania site, "Bioethics for Beginners."

III. Thought and Discussion

- What information about yourself do you consider private? Financial? Medical?
- If you give information to one person or company, do they have the right to share it with others? If so, under what conditions? If not, why not?
- Should an action related to information (such as breaching confidentiality) be given the same moral weight as a physical act against another person (such as assault)?
- If you examine a patient in another state by using a two-way video, what are the implications in terms of licensure, privacy, confidentiality, and scope of practice?

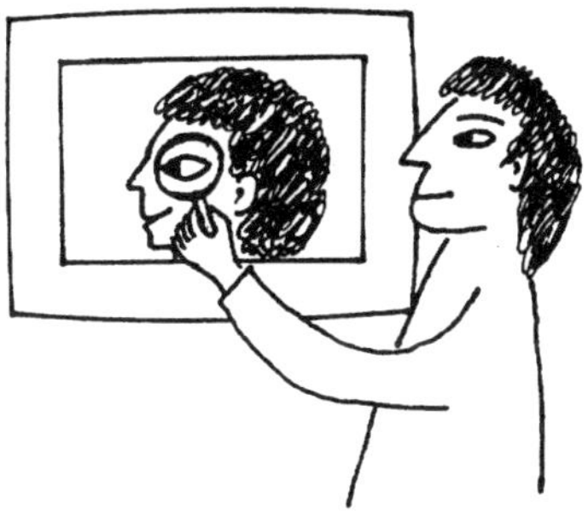

- What ethical issues are relevant to your field? Name five specific dilemmas that you face every day at work.

Readings From the Net

(Links available at http://NewWindPub.com/workbook)

Ethics

Maclean Center for Clinical Medical Ethics	http://ccme-mac4.bsd.uchicago.edu	Interdisciplinary group at the University of Chicago.
MedWeb bioethics resources	http://www.gen.emory.edu/medweb/medweb.bioethics.html	Documents, guidelines, publications, Internet resources, societies. Long list.
The Net: User Guidelines and Netiquette	http://www.fau.edu/rinaldi/net	Set of ethical guidelines for the many different kinds of electronic communication and transaction: email, discussion groups, WWW, moving files.
UB Center for Clinical Ethics	http://wings.buffalo.edu/faculty/research/bioethics/other.html	Organizations, societies.

Copyright

Copyright Act of 1976	http://www.law.cornell.edu/uscode/17	Full text of the Act.
The Copyright Question	http://www.iw.com/1997/01/ copyright.html	Article from Internet World, linking to several online sources.
The Copyright Website	http://www.benedict.com	News, source documents, books.
Creative Incentive Coalition	http://www.cic.org	Working to maintain copyright.
U.S. Copyright Office	http://lcweb.loc.gov/copyright	Official info, forms, basics.

Privacy

Electronic Frontier Foundation (EFF)	http://www.eff.org	Well-known organization founded by John Barlow.
Electronic Privacy Information Center	http://www.epic.org	News, resources, extensive archive of articles.
Internet Privacy Coalition	http://www.privacy.org/ipc	Resources, chronology, alerts.

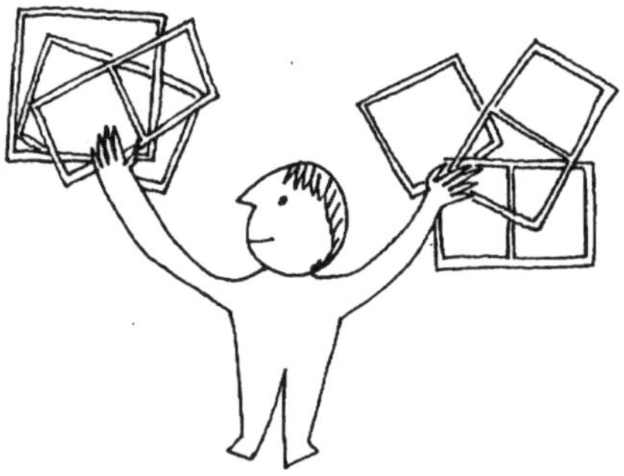

Chapter 14: Mailing Lists, Discussion Groups

The Moving Finger writes; and, having writ,
Moves on: nor all thy Piety nor Wit
Shall lure it back to cancel half a Line,
Nor all thy Tears wash out a Word of it.
The Rubáiyát of Omar Khayyam
trans., *Edward Fitzgerald*

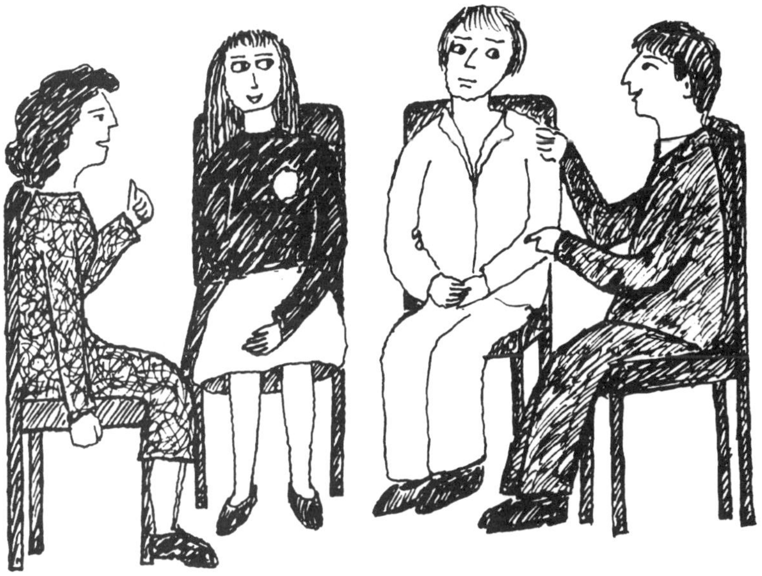

IN THIS CHAPTER

archive
articles
closed, open list
digest
discussion group
hierarchies
listserv, listproc
mailing list
marking
moderator
newsgroup
posting
subscribing
thread

Introduction

Mailing lists and newsgroups are simple but powerful tools of communication. A single message often reverberates through a hundred email boxes, or travels around the world via a newsgroup. In the realm of information you see the "butterfly effect" every day, where a small initial message causes large and unpredictable results.

Mailing lists

A mailing list is a means for any number of people to send messages to each other. When you "subscribe" to a list (by sending an email message to the computer which runs it) the computer puts your email address on the list. Then every time that someone sends a message to the list, you receive a copy.

Some lists are completely automatic. Subscribing, unsubscribing, asking for help are all done by a program called Listserv or Listproc. Other lists can have some degree of human supervision. The moderator of the list may want to control who can subscribe, or which messages can be sent to the list. Computer programs which run lists allow for different degrees of automation.

Subscribing to a mailing list is free. To subscribe, you send a message to the computer running the list. (Don't send the message to the list itself, which is a common mistake.) For example, if Mary Doe wants to subscribe to a list called Health-L run by listserv@computer.com, she sends a message to listserv@computer.com and in the body of the message, types subscribe Health-L Mary Doe To unsubscribe, she follows the same procedure but uses the word unsubscribe instead.

When you subscribe to a list, the listserv computer will send a confirmation message back to you. This message will also tell you how to unsubscribe, and usually gives a brief introduction to the purpose of the list. It's a good idea to create a folder in your email program to save messages from the list.

In our example, when Mary wants to send a message to the people on the list, she uses the address Health-L@computer.com She will know that the list is working because as a member she will get a copy of her own message.

Archive

A collection of past information or records.

Many lists put all messages sent into an archive. You can search these archives to see what past conversations have been about, or use the archive to find a message that you have deleted.

Although most people who subscribe to lists simply use them to send and receive messages, the program which runs the list can do many other things: provide a list of the members, unsubscribe you while you are on vacation, tell you more about the program itself, or send you messages in a batch rather than one at a time. Here are some examples of commands that you use to accomplish these tasks.

Common mistake

Sending a command to the list rather than the computer.

You send commands to the computer (e.g. listserv@computer.com) and <u>not</u> to the list itself (e.g. Health-L@computer.com). When sending a command, don't put anything in the subject line, and turn off your signature if you have one. Send only one command per message. In the examples below, *listname* would be the name of the list, for example Health-L.

information *listname*	Sends an introduction to that specific list.
help	Sends a help document about these commands.
review *listname*	Sends you a list and address for each member.
set *listname* ***conceal***	Hides you from others using the review command.
set *listname* ***digest***	Mail is distributed to you in a batch (usually weekly).
set *listname* ***nomail***	Mail delivery will be stopped, if you are on vacation.
set *listname* ***mail***	Starts delivery again.

Information Overload

Beware of joining several mailing lists. The number of email messages you receive can add up to dozens or even hundreds a day. It can be difficult just to read and think about a quiet list which exchanges only a few messages. I recently spoke to someone who told me he has subscribed to so many lists that he gets 1,500 messages a day! If that happens, you are already drowning in the ocean of information.

What a List Can Accomplish

Why should you join a mailing list? Here are some ways a list can be helpful.

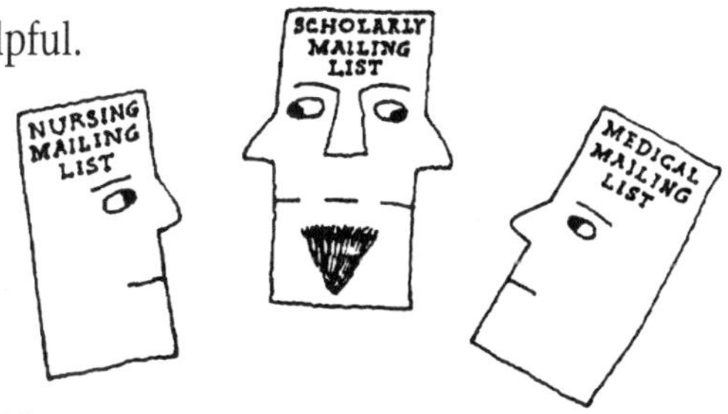

- students in a class can ask each other questions or exchange notes
- teachers can send out assignments, notes, or grades
- work groups can manage projects, drafts, meetings
- departments can send memos and notices
- clinicians can discuss a specific topic or specialty
- patients and families with a specific condition can support each other
- companies can send out updates about products

Finding Mailing Lists

There are more than 50,000 mailing lists operating on the Internet. They range from lists limited to ten students in one class, to worldwide lists with hundreds of subscribers. The quickest way to find a mailing list in your specialty may be to go to a Web site for that specialty. In addition to links, these sites often contain descriptions and addresses for mailing lists.

Another way is to look in a subject directory or search engine for mailing lists. These will include lists of every type and description, so you may have to look around until you find what you need. Tile.net (http://www.tile.net/tile/listserv) lets you look up lists by description, name, subject, country, and organization.

Usenet Newsgroups

You are probably familiar with bulletin boards in a library. A person puts up a note ("Why do the lights go out 15 minutes before closing time?" is a favorite) and later a librarian posts a reply. Newsgroups work much the same way, except that the bulletin board is on the Internet, and anyone in the world can read a note or reply to it!

For example, you send a message to a group devoted to AIDS, asking about new drug therapies. Someone reads your note and sends a reply. Another person sends a note correcting something you wrote. And the discussion goes on.

> *Hierarchy*
>
> A system of classification.

The entire collection of bulletin boards, called Usenet, is organized into subjects, each of which has an abbreviation. Examples of subjects ("hierarchies") are science (sci), recreation (rec), miscellaneous (misc) or computer (comp). The name of a newsgroup is an abbreviated description. Look at the name sci.med.nursing. It is in the general category of science (sci), in the medical area (med), covering nursing. Within a hierarchy there may be hundreds or thousands of groups. Today there are more than 15,000 different Usenet groups.

Think of a newsgroup as an ongoing conversation taking place in a large room. When you open a newsgroup on your computer, the conversation has already been going on for some time, and you will probably see hundreds of messages.

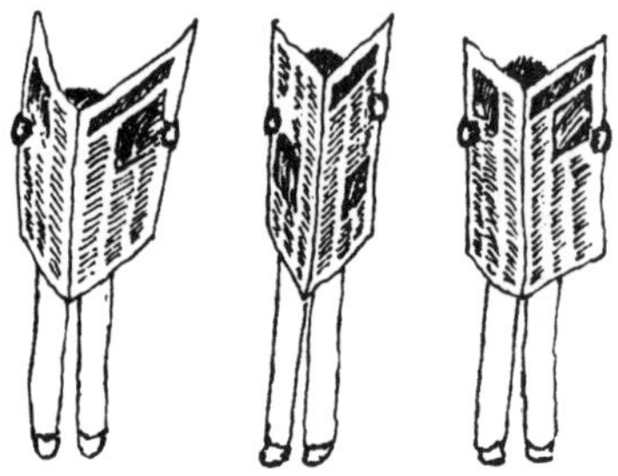

Posting a Message

When you read a message, you can respond to the entire group or to the person who sent it, or both. If you send a message to the newsgroup, it may be read by dozens or thousands of others, some of whom may respond. A message stays on the news server for a few weeks, and then is erased to make room for new ones. (Technically, your message is sent to the local news server, which then sends it to another group of servers, and so on until it has gone around the world.)

Subscribing to a Newsgroup

Thread

A series of messages on a newsgroup about a particular topic.

Subscribing to a newsgroup is free. When you subscribe to a newsgroup, Netscape (or your news reader program) adds the name of the group to a file on your computer. There is no money involved, and unlike a mailing list, nobody else knows that you have subscribed.

When you are looking at the messages in a particular group, the program will arrange messages into threads of discussion. When one person sends a comment and several persons respond, that is one thread of discussion.

Finding Newsgroups

Finding newsgroups is getting easier. Netscape 4 includes a searchable list that is compiled from the news server. You can also find lists and descriptions of newsgroups on the Web.

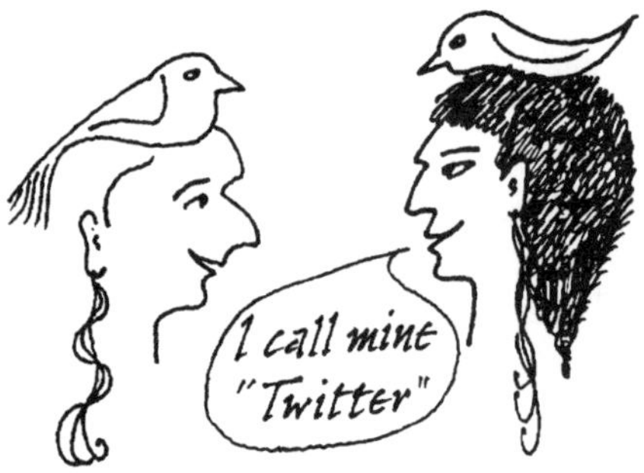

Moderated, Edited, Free-for-All

The Usenet is a good way to communicate with other people who are interested in a topic. You can read and exchange messages every day, and I guarantee that you will find somebody who shares your interest, no matter how odd, transient, or flighty it may be.

Remember that most messages that are posted to Usenet are not edited or moderated. As a source of authoritative information on a topic, Usenet is not very reliable. The Net is rife with false information, half-truths, urban myths, and lots and lots and lots of questions.

When messages to a group are moderated the quality of discussion is significantly improved. There are also fewer messages because the moderator must review each one before posting it.

Setting up Netscape to Read Newsgroups

Netscape includes a program for reading newsgroups and posting messages to them. In order to use it, you have to set up Netscape so it will connect to a news computer (server) that carries the messages. See the exercises at the end of Chapter 5 if you need to do this.

EXERCISES

Each lettered exercise is independent.
(Links available at http://NewWindPub.com/workbook)

I. Guided Practice

A. OPEN A NEWSGROUP

If you are not familiar with Netscape's email window, go back to Chapter 5 and work through those exercises now. Netscape uses its email program to send messages to newsgroups.

1. Click in the location bar to highlight the entire address.
2. Type `news:sci.med.nursing`
3. Press the Enter key.
4. Netscape will open a separate newsgroup window. (Netscape 3: You will see three rectangular areas (frames). One shows the news computer (server) and the name of the group (sci.med.nursing). The other shows the messages that you can read. The third window displays each individual message.) (Netscape 4: You will see two rectangular areas (frames). The top one shows the messages that you can read, and the bottom one displays each individual message.)
5. Click a message to see it.
6. The borders between each rectangular window can be moved to make reading easier. Click a border and drag it to resize the windows.
7. Note that some messages have a minus (-) sign next to them. This means that someone has answered the message, starting a "thread" of discussion.
8. Click a minus (-) sign to expand the thread of messages.
9. Click a plus (+) sign to contract a thread of messages.

OPEN A SECOND NEWSGROUP FOR PRACTICE IN SENDING MESSAGES

1. Click the File, Add Newsgroup menu.
2. Type `misc.test` and press the Enter key.
3. (Netscape 4: Type `news:misc.test` and press the Enter key.)
4. Post a message to the newsgroup
5. Click File, New News Message or the button which says To: news (Netscape 4: File, New, Message)
6. An email window opens, with the message addressed to the group misc.test
7. Type `ignore` in the subject line, and `this is a test` in the body of the message.
8. Click the Send button.

II. Problem-Solving

- Find a mailing list in your specialty (use Chapter 12) and subscribe to it for a couple of weeks.
- Use Liszt (http://www.liszt.com) to find a mailing list and request automated information from the list without subscribing.

III. Thought and Discussion

- Explain what "many-to-many" means in terms of newsgroups.
- Suppose your coworkers or fellow students have access to the Internet and email. How can you use a newsgroup or mailing list to help each other?
- Imagine that someone has just written a scathing personal comment about you to a mailing list. What would you do? What if you were the moderator of the list?
- The word "noise" has been used to describe the huge amount of irrelevant information on the Usenet, which can make it difficult to find something useful. Discuss ways to decrease the "noise" in a clinical setting.

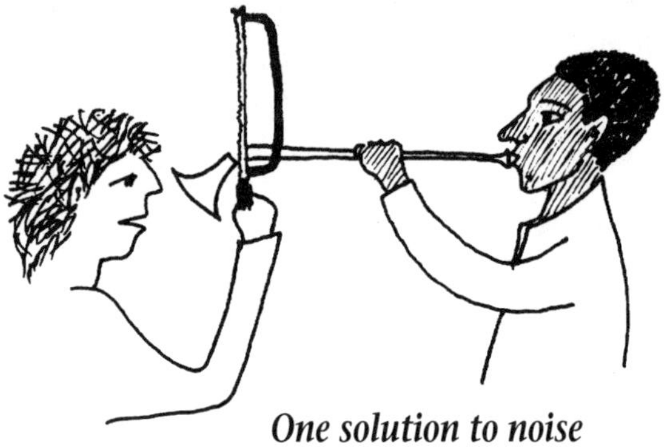

One solution to noise

Links and Readings from the Net

Newsgroups

(Links available at http://NewWindPub.com/workbook)

AltaVista	http://www.altavista.digital.com	Searches articles for a word or phrase.
FAQ's	http://www.cis.ohio-state.edu/hypertext/faq/usenet/top.html	FAQ's for all newsgroups listed in news.answers.
DejaNews	http://www.dejanews.com	Searches articles; retrieves an entire thread.
Liszt	http://www.liszt.com	Searchable list of newsgroups.
Oxford	http://www.lib.ox.ac.uk/internet/news	Annotated list of groups.
Usenet Archive	http://www.netannounce.org	Newsgroup to introduce Usenet.
Usenet Help	http://sunsite.unc.edu/usenet-i	General and technical info.

Mailing Lists

Liszt	http://www.liszt.com	Searchable list of lists.
Mailing lists	http://ifrit.web.aol.com/mld/production	Well organized, easy to read.
Mailing lists	http://www.nlc-bnc.ca/ifla/I/training/listserv/lists.htm	Introduction and links to documents and guides.
Mailing lists	http://www.nova.edu/Inter-Links/listserv.html	Searchable directory and how-to guides.

Chapter 15: Managing Time and Information

Today, the materials and skills from which a life is composed are no longer clear. It is no longer possible to follow the paths of previous generations.

Mary Catherine Bateson, Composing a Life

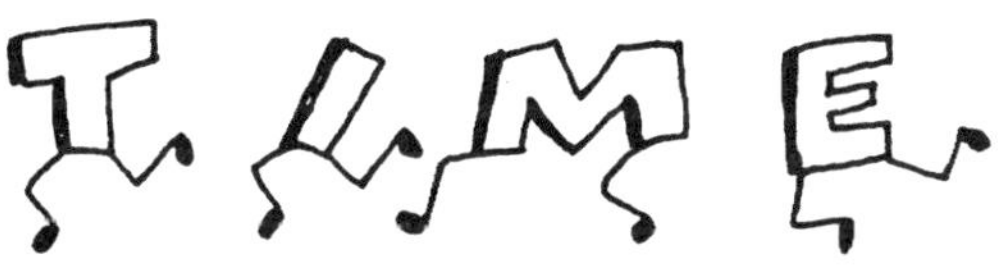

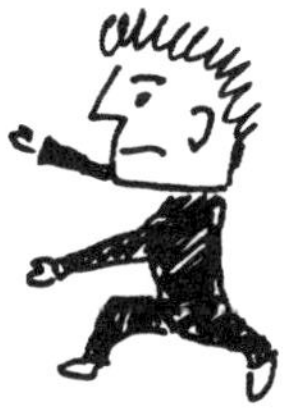

IN THIS CHAPTER

daybook
fluency
follow-up
interoffice mail
jargon
notebook
pager
telemedicine
voice mail

Life is different than it was fifty or even twenty years ago. Knowledge is accumulating faster; news of local or world events reaches us sooner; people change jobs several times during a single decade. In one day as a professional you are likely to have several discussions with others about fundamental issues; make appointments for meetings in the coming weeks and months; write several pages of notes; answer multiple telephone calls or voice mail messages; and look up facts on a handful of conditions and treatments. Then you will go home, read the paper, and watch the news. By this point, most of us start having memory-buffer congestion problems, unless, like Shrödinger's cat, we can be in two or three places at once.

New information technologies do not save time, they enable us to engage in more and different activities. In today's technojargon, we are multitasking, spending smaller slices of time on more projects. If we use technology well we will be that much more productive, but it is easy to be drowned by an ever-rising tide of information.

Voice communication

Respond Immediately

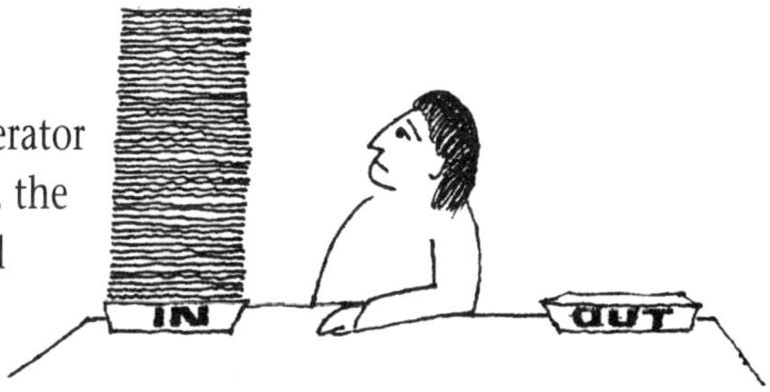

What do you think when a physician doesn't answer his pager, or an operator doesn't answer the phone? Whether it be a call bell, voice mail, or email, the single most important quality of a response, and the one that people will remember, is speed. If necessary, the information can be found later.

Waiting half an hour to respond to a call bell is too long, just as waiting a week is too long to respond to voice mail. I know a manager who doesn't answer her voice mail or email for weeks at a time, and her reputation has been harmed irreparably. When you fail to answer, people will assume that you're overwhelmed by your job, you're lazy, or you just don't care about their concerns. Think about it.

Make Instant Decisions

Voice mail and email are often used to send rapid messages: Can you come today? Did you hear about this report? What do you think about this article? Always send back a quick answer, then delete the message. If you save every message in order to think about it later, you will never read any of them, much less respond.

Slow Down for Important Discussions

Although you should respond to simple requests immediately, take a few hours or a day to respond to the more important or emotional questions. Many people get into trouble because they send out voice mail or email in the heat of the moment without considering what they are saying or how they are expressing themselves. If you feel worked up when composing a message, save it for at least twenty-four hours. Always. If you still want to send it after that period, fine. But you will be surprised how many times you will change your mind after a good night's sleep.

Learn to Summarize

When you page a physician, be prepared to give a one-minute history, assessment, and recommendation. How many nurses call up a physician and say "Oh, doctor? What do you think about the bleeding?" If you don't give a physician the necessary information, you turn your conversation into a guessing game. "What patient? What problem are we discussing? What medication is she taking?"

Jargon

The technical terms used in a profession.

Summarizing is a skill that takes time and practice to learn, but after you have mastered the technique you can use it everywhere. Shift report, staff meetings, voice mail, email, conference presentations, talks with your family are all situations where you will be more effective (and they will be happier) if you can marshal your ideas and present them in a brief, logical order. "Hi, this is Jane from dietary. Did you know that Mr. X is on a low salt diet when you wrote the order for pretzels? Please get back to me before eleven, when lunch is served. You can reach me on beeper 1234."

Know When to Translate Your Jargon

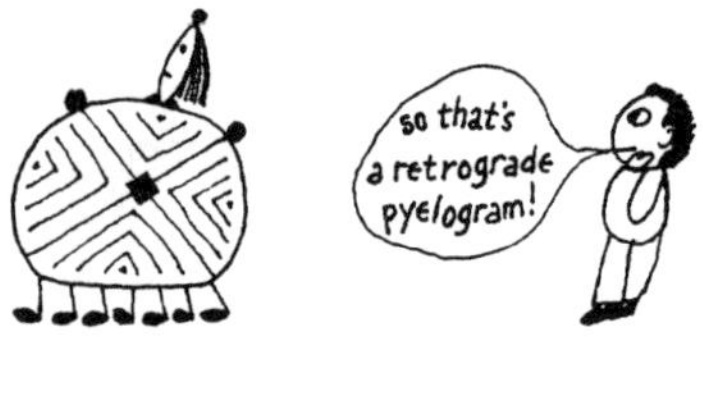

Technical jargon allows persons in a profession to communicate in a kind of mental shorthand. "Cancel that CT on Mrs. Y. Her lytes are out of balance; I want to do a chem panel first." Talking like this to other professionals is appropriate and necessary in every field. But don't be so much in love with technical words that you forget to translate when talking to others. The measure of your intelligence is not the jargon you know, but your ability to set it aside when necessary. If you're really intelligent, you can explain a retrograde pyelogram to a five-year old.

Machine Culture: Pick Your Tools

Different jobs require different tools, including information tools. Just because a technology is available doesn't mean that you should use it. Yet deciding whether to use a tool is a pragmatic decision, not a Faustian bargain with your soul. Email simply doesn't help in a code blue, any more than a pager helps in an English class. The first question you must ask yourself is, "Why do I need a (voice mail box, fax, email address, Web page)?"

Pager

Expected response time: fifteen minutes. The only reason to have a pager is to be available in emergencies. If you sit in one office all day, or work in one clinic, a pager is unnecessary: people will call you. If you do have one, respond to pages in fifteen minutes, unless you're asleep, bicycling, or in the middle of a code, in which case you get an extra ten minutes...

Voice Mail

Expected response time: same work day. Voice mail is the equivalent of other kinds of mail: you get a box where people can leave messages. They can often address the message to you by name rather than by telephone number. Messages can be saved or forwarded to other people. You can make good use of voice mail if you work in a large institution and need to communicate with many people. A person can leave you a quick message, which you answer later in the day.

Email

Expected response time: one to two days. Email is useful for managers, educators, planners, and others who generate documents or coordinate teams of people. It is also extremely useful for communicating with professionals in other states or countries. However, email causes problems for many people right now, for several reasons.

If you are part of a large organization, you may easily get more email messages than phone calls. It is common to have between five and twenty messages every day. Reading and answering these can take an hour or more.

Managers who can't type are in a difficult situation. Personal secretaries have become a thing of the past for middle management, yet managers are expected to perform the same tasks as they did before (comment upon, revise, or generate documents). For a slow typist, answering even a simple email may seem like an intrusion on other, more important work. A manager may be hesitant to admit she lacks the necessary typing skill, or unwilling to take the time to learn. (Inexpensive or free typing programs are available, with exercises, tests, and tutorials, so you can learn at home on your computer.)

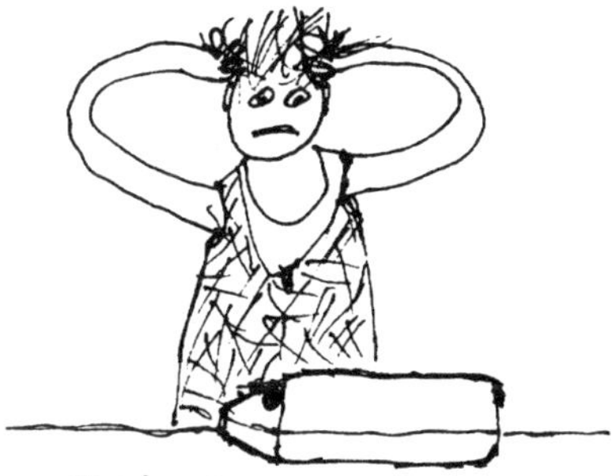

Typing trauma

Email is still used ineffectively by many people, which creates barriers to communication rather than overcoming them. Quoting the entire text of the message you are responding to, rather than just the relevant passages, forces the person reading it to scroll past or skim a long message before even seeing your response.

Because it is still new, many people are excited when they discover they can send email to a niece in Iowa or a friend in Germany. They spend more time on personal than work-related correspondence. Then managers want to take away email privileges. Work when you work, and play when you play. Don't mix the two.

Web Site

"When I found so astonishing a power placed within my hands, I hesitated a long time concerning the manner in which I should employ it." (Mary Wollstonecraft Shelley, *Frankenstein*) Do you need a Web site? Will it help your work? Unless you can answer yes to all of the following questions, the Web is probably not the best choice for you at this time.

- Are you responsible for a set of documents which people rely upon (policies, manuals, handouts) or those which need to be continually updated (phone book, on-call list)?

- Do you have the personnel necessary to convert the documents to Web format?

- Does your organization have a functioning Web site supported by an available technical staff?

Telemedicine

Practicing medicine at a distance.

Telemedicine Link

Although still in its early stages, telemedicine on the horizon. If you are a physician in a rural clinic and you often perform procedures where a specialist would be useful, you may want to check with your parent organization or the nearest university hospital. They may have a telemedicine program you can join.

Simple Solutions

Notebook

Thoughts come and go in a few seconds. You'll be surprised how useful a little external memory is. "Since the time I was a young man, I have always kept a notebook handy when I read a book." (Akira Kurosawa) Every conscientious writer carries a notebook at all times to jot down an idea, whether it occurs on the freeway, in the middle of a phone conversation, or walking by the river.

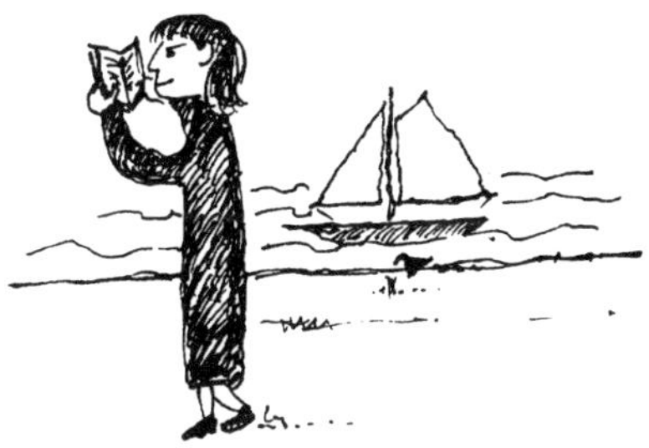

For the first two years after I started working as a nurse I kept a little pocket notebook for writing down all the peculiar bits of knowledge, procedures, or persons that came my way. One day I sat down and organized them into categories, and suddenly we had an orientation manual.

Filing Cabinet

If you are a health professional, and especially if you have ambitions of moving into teaching or management, you need a filing cabinet for the surfeit of papers that are likely to pass through your hands. For a few dollars you can get a cardboard version, just to try out the idea. Then look through the stacks of paper that are sitting around on your desk, or on your clipboard, and see how they can be categorized. For each category, create a file folder.

Every five years go through your cabinet and throw out materials you don't need, to keep from accumulating useless paper.

Daybook

A daybook is a pocket-sized calendar where you write down your appointments for each day. For a staff nurse, a daybook isn't of much use, but for a manager it is essential. Use a book that you can keep with you at all times: you will find people asking to set up meetings in the elevator, at lunch, even in the supermarket.

Interoffice Mail

Keep a stack of re-mailers (the envelopes which have multiple lines on them, for sending over and over) in your desk. Then, whenever someone asks for a document, toss it into an envelope. The next time you go to the mail room, take the mail of the day with you to drop off.

Advanced Skills

Concentration

Most tasks can be done in a fraction of the time, if we would simply concentrate. Learning how to focus your mind can open up new careers, enable you to have more interesting hobbies, let you learn a second language, even transform your life. Concentration will give you more time, because those tasks which used to take several hours can now be done in minutes.

> *Fluency*
>
> The ability to write quickly and accurately.

Fluency In Speech and Writing

Many people think that writing is a skill a person is born with. Nothing could be further from the truth. We all learn to speak and write, and we can teach ourselves better methods even in middle age. If you would like to be able to write well but it takes you half an hour to write a three-sentence memo, read *Becoming a Writer* (Brande, 1934).

Grokking the Gestalt

Cultivate the ability to walk onto your unit and in ten seconds see the entire situation: how busy the shift is likely to be, whether the previous staff are overstressed, how the patients are doing. For this you will need some insight into human nature, a dash of intuition, and attention to detail.

Running a Meeting

Running a meeting involves a combination of emotional insight, mental concentration, and just plain luck. "Talent develops in quiet places, character in the full current of human life." (Goethe) If your staff meetings are out of control, set up strict guidelines, such as *Robert's Rules of Order*. If your meetings never seem to result in anything, end each of them with a plan for action: who is going to do what and when. If you can never get through all the issues, hold your meetings more often.

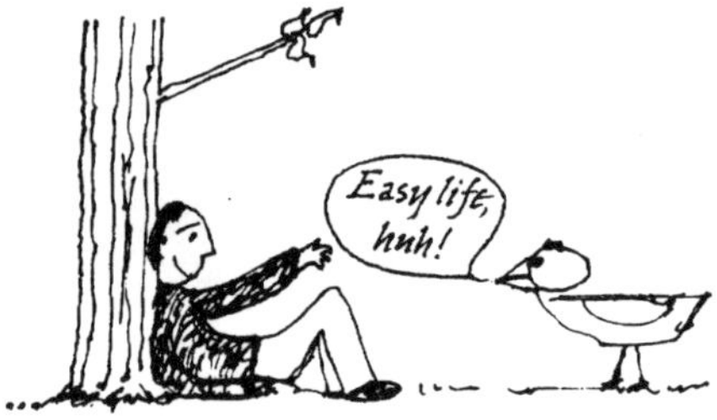

Relaxation

It may seem odd to include relaxation as an advanced skill, but very few people know how to relax. Getting drunk, arguing with your spouse, or working at a second job does not relax the body or the mind. Instead, try to laugh, get outside the building for a few minutes, lie down in a dark room, play with your cat, or take a hot shower. You don't need a course in zazen or TM; just close your eyes and breathe deep.

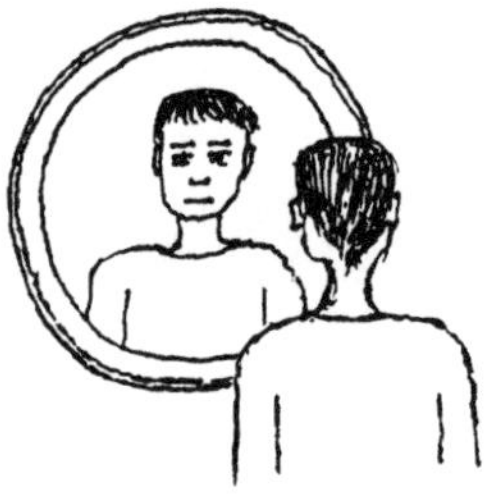

Self Observation

Observe yourself at work. Do you complain all the time, snap at coworkers, spin your wheels while trying to decide what to do, blame others for your problems? Do people seek you out, or do they avoid you? Do people talk to you about the ideas they are having? If you know your true character, you will be better at your job, no matter what your profession.

Putting it all Together

Every form of communication has different connotations, different nuances. Personal problems are better dealt with face to face. Voice mail and email are good for issues. Faxes tend to be seen by someone other than the recipient, and so should not be used for private correspondence.

Many people prefer one form of communication over another. One manager may detest email, but love to receive faxes. Another may dislike both, and prefer to do everything over the phone. Be flexible: communicate with people in the form they feel comfortable with. As long as the message is sent, or the work gets done, the medium makes no difference at all.

EXERCISES

Each lettered exercise is independent.

II. Problem-Solving

- Walk around your unit for ten minutes, then write down a list by topic of all the information resources available.
- Break up into groups of three. Pick a topic, and have two people present a different viewpoint. Then have the third person summarize the two viewpoints and suggest a compromise.
- Pick an ongoing problem on your unit or at school. Break into groups of five and appoint a chairperson for each group. As the chair, actively moderate and lead the discussion so that in half an hour you have a written solution that reflects the consensus of the group.
- Buy a small notebook that will fit in your pocket. For three days, write down every new piece of information as you learn it.
- Take two minutes to think about it, then present a 30-second summary of everything you did today.

III. Thought and Discussion

- How did the Democratic party use organizational techniques related to information in the national election of 1996?
- What different mental skills are necessary for these tasks: taking a patient history, sorting through differential diagnoses, writing a physical assessment, and reading an EKG?

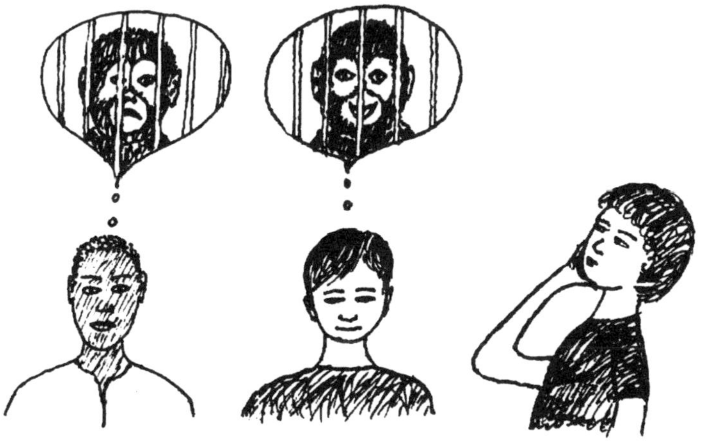

Compromise and consensus

Chapter 16: Troubleshooting

Experience is the name everyone gives to their mistakes.

Oscar Wilde

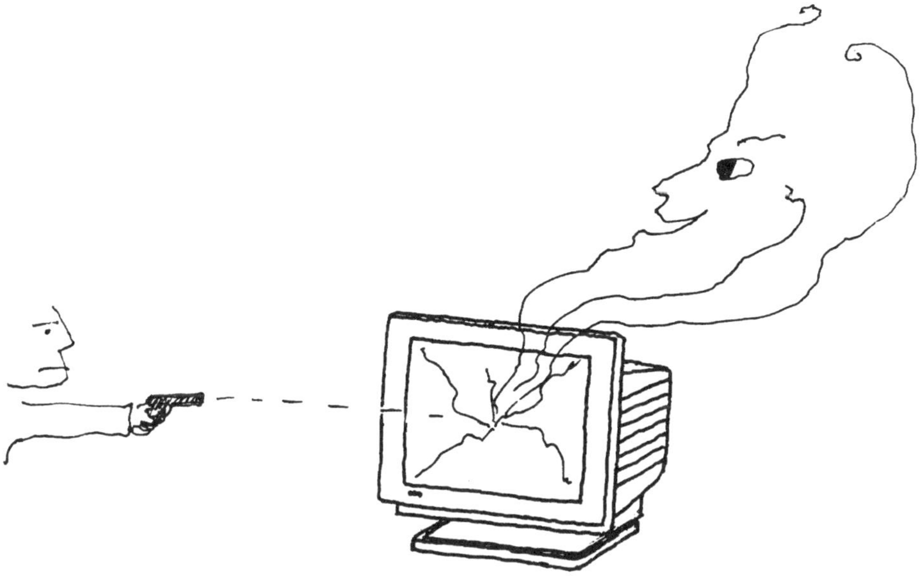

IN THIS CHAPTER

backup
cfgback.exe
defragment
error messages
eru.exe
re-boot
registry
scandisk
startup disk
viruses

General principles

Computers have lots of problems

Expect problems, especially when installing new equipment or programs. Modern computers and the Microsoft Windows operating system display what a physicist might call quantum weirdness. If you don't take some elementary precautions, someday your work may end up in that big bit bucket in the sky.

Re-boot First

When computers start, they use their own program, a process that is likened to pulling itself up by its own bootstraps. Hence the phrase to "boot" a computer. "Re-booting" means to re-start the computer. Don't use your L.L. Bean clodhoppers.

Computers get themselves tied up in data knots more often than you would think. Many problems are solved by re-booting (Ctrl+Alt+Del keys), using the Reset button, or turning the power off and re-starting the computer after fifteen seconds. Re-booting is often the solution when a program gets instant Parkinson's, or your little rodent develops drunk mouse syndrome. If a computer doesn't start, a start-up disk may be needed. See the exercises for instructions on creating a start-up disk.

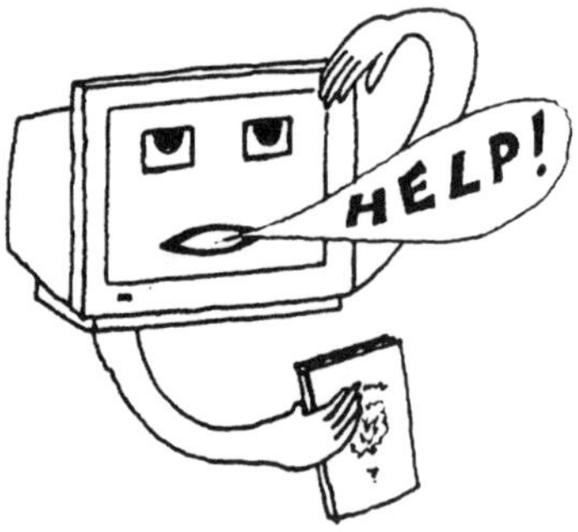

People are your best resource - not books

Trying random actions to solve a problem when you know absolutely nothing often makes things worse, or at the very least will waste your time. It's okay to solve problems you understand, but know your limitations. When you need help, people are your best resource. As you gain experience, books and online documents become more useful.

Work from simple to complex

Don't assume every technical challenge is a zebra. Just as with human disease, most computer problems are common and well-known, and have simple solutions. If you can't print a Web page, check the printer first. Is it plugged in? Turned on? See if you can print from a small program such as Notepad. Finally, check the settings in the program you are using.

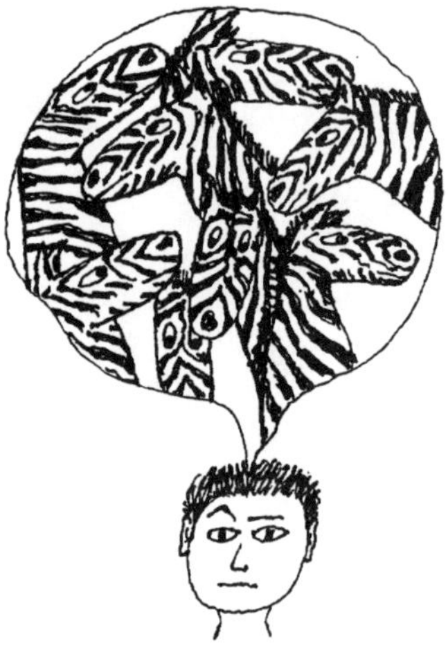

Zebras on my mind

My coworker recently bought a new piece of hardware for her home computer and promptly got into a state of total wedgitude trying to get it to work. She spent forty hours testing everything: cables, interrupts, other cards, memory. Then a friend came over, plugged the card into another slot, and it worked fine.

Richard Feynman, one of the most original minds of our time, wrote "We must remove the rigidity of thought...We must have freedom for the mind to wander about in trying to solve... problems."

Review the history of the disease

History is just as important in diagnosing and solving technical problems as it is with health care, whether you are doing the work yourself or calling for help. Did the problem occur when:

- you turned on the computer?
- you logged in?
- Windows was starting?
- Netscape or Explorer was starting?
- you downloaded a file?
- the lights went out for a second?
- you loaded a new program?

Write down error messages if you don't understand them

Technical people and los hardwaristas can only help if they know what went wrong. Fatal error? General protection fault? System on siesta? Remembering to write down these messages takes some time to learn, but get into the habit of taking notes.

Know the name of the program you are using

Word? Word Perfect? Excel? Technical people can't help you if they don't know what you are using, just as a physician can't give advice about "somebody in the

ICU." Many computer books advise you to know everything about your computer, including CPU, memory, operating system. That's often unnecessary, but at the very least be able to give the name of the program. Who knows, someday you may be face to face with Gort, and the fate of the world will depend on remembering "Klaatu barada nikto."

Prevention is better than cure

Everyone has computer problems. Everyone. The question is how severe they will be, and how difficult it will be to return to normal. A few simple precautions will save you days, even weeks of grief. DO ALL OF THE FOLLOWING AS SOON AS YOU CAN!

> ***Startup Disk***
>
> A floppy disk that can be used to start a computer.

1. Make a startup disk. This is a floppy disk that enables you to start the computer if something is drastically wrong with the operating system and it can't start itself.
2. (Windows 95) Run the eru.exe and cfgback.exe programs. Run the cfgback.exe program again before you add each new program. See the Guided Exercises below for instructions on running these two programs.
3. Backup all important information to a physically separate disk or tape as often as you think necessary. This can be done with a floppy, once a day or once every few months. It all depends on how often the information changes, and how important it is to have a fool-proof copy.
4. Install, learn to use, and keep the files current on a good anti-virus program.
5. Defragment your hard drive at least once every six months.
6. Check every new floppy and program for viruses, including those purchased in a store or downloaded from major computer sites. Never leave floppies in the drive when you turn off your computer, so that boot viruses won't get a chance to infect your computer.

Helping Other People Solve Computer Problems

Be calm, cheerful, and confident

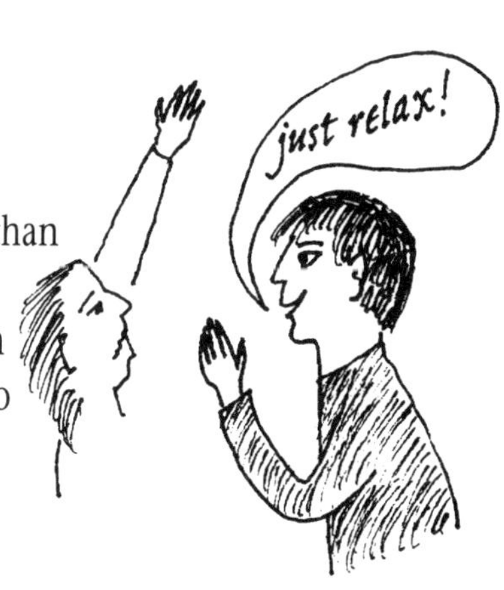

Your attitude toward a person having a computer problem is more important than any technical knowledge you may have. He may be facing the Black Screen of Death for the first time, and be (understandably) a trifle anxious. Reassure him that you will be able to help, if you think you can, or that you will refer him to the right technical department.

Gently take charge

Unless you really want to listen to yet another half-hour diatribe about shoddy Microsoft products, turn the conversation fairly soon to the problem at hand. Be supportive but specific. Try to determine as soon as you can if this is a problem you can solve, or whether it's a mandelbug that technical support needs to look at.

Backtrack

Talk the person back to the beginning of the problem, and then go forward. How did the problem begin? How important is it? How soon does it need to be solved? If he can't print, has he ever been able to? If the computer is running slowly, how long has it been happening?

Some problems, such as the fact that the person is using a 386 and everyone else has a Pentium, do not have quick or simple solutions.

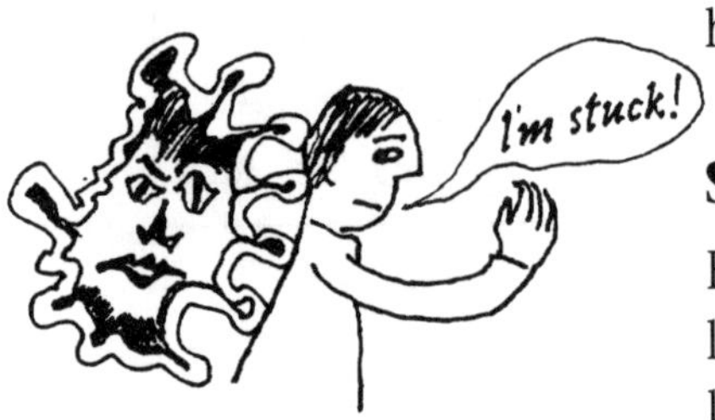

Stick to the immediate problem

Because it is so difficult to find anyone who will truly help with computers, at any level, the other person may well start asking about other things. How do I download files from the Internet? Will I get a virus if I take a disk home? Be supportive, but don't get coerced into a complete brain dump.

Solve it, don't refer the person to a manual

Nothing is more frustrating to a busy person than to be told "Oh, that's simple. Just look in the (thousand-page) Windows resource kit." If you have the knowledge, either talk him through it on the phone or solve it in person. As a last resort, send detailed, step-by-step instructions. Anything less is no solution at all. This applies to situations you might not think of as problems, such as "How do I create two columns in Word Perfect?" If a person can't get the work done, it's a problem.

Step-by-step approach to troubleshooting

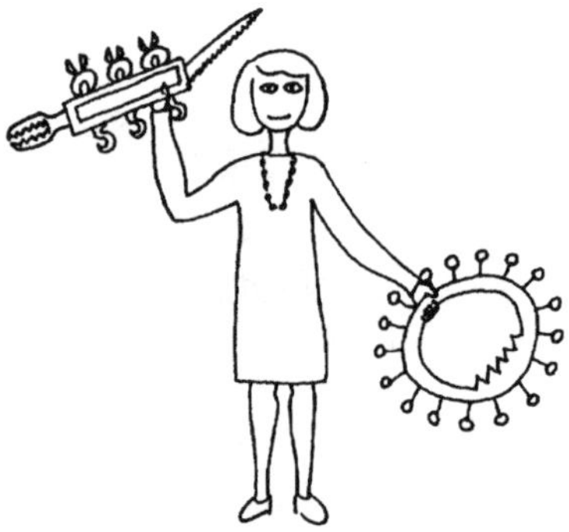

1. Find out what the problem is. Get a good history.
2. Go back to the basics. Try all the plugs. Re-boot.
3. Check for changes. New program?
4. Run the program. Re-create the situation.
5. Run scandisk and defrag. Fix lost clusters and cross-linked files.
6. Look on the company's Web site for updates, new drivers, notes about incompatibility.
7. Call somebody who knows more than you do.

The following table is meant to help you diagnose some common problems. These are starting points; for most of these you will need additional information than is given below. A good place to start is the Help menu of the program you are using.

Getting Started

Problem	*Possible Solution*
Computer is slow	Check the turbo switch. Check for permanent swap file enabled (Windows 3.1). Check that hard drive has at least 10 MB free space. Check for 32-bit file access (Windows 3.1). Defragment hard drive. Delete temporary (*.tmp) files. Use a smaller program to accomplish the task. Buy a new computer.
Can't connect to the Internet	Make sure modem is plugged in and attached. Check that line is in the correct jack in the modem. Make sure correct software drives are installed for that modem. Install Dialup Networking (Windows 95). Check service provider phone number. Check Control Panel/Network for client (Windows 95). Make sure you are using TCP/IP (Control Panel/Network).

Email

Problem	*Possible Solution*
Can't send mail	Check preferences for server and identity. Check outbox for mail that is queued up but unable to go. Check addressbook to see if address was entered correctly.
Mail returns to me	Check spelling of address you are sending to. Check if person's mailing address has changed.
Attachments won't open	Check file name of attachment. See if you have the same program used to create the file. Check with the person who sent it to see if he is using Unix or Macintosh. Get program to convert attachments if necessary. Open word processor, then open the attachment from within program.
Can't send an attachment	Check to see if file is open in another program.
Incoming attachments have problems	May need to reinstall mail program or initialization file.
Inbox messages are in a strange order	Click the header of the Date column to arrange messages by date.
Messages are printed with odd line breaks	Check Settings/Fonts. Make sure that screen and print font are the same.
When I send to a list I've created, each recipient sees everyone else's address	When sending, use Bcc: instead of To: or Cc:
Message was open, now it's lost	Check Window menu. Message window may be minimized or behind another window.

Browsing the Web

Problem	*Possible Solution*
Nothing happens	Check network or modem connection. Close browser and re-boot.
Everything is slow	Upgrade to a faster modem. Upgrade to Windows 95. Browse during the morning or late evening. Turn off automatic loading of images.
Bookmarks disappear	Check with network administrator on Netscape configuration.
Error message	See http://www.cnet.com/Resources/Tech/Advisers/Error
400 Bad Request	Make sure you typed the URL correctly.
401 Authorization Required	Ask Webmaster for password or other restrictions.
403 Forbidden	Ask Webmaster for password or other restrictions.
404 Not found	Check your typing. Page may have moved. Go one level up.
500 Server error	Webserver glitch. Email the Webmaster if you need that page.
503 Service Unavailable	Try again later. Server or network may not be working.
Connection Refused by Host	Ask Webmaster for password or other restrictions.
Host Unknown	Check your typing. Try later. Server may not be working.
Can't see video, animation	Get plug-in (http://home.netscape.com).Download full version of Netscape.

Searching

No results found	Check your spelling. Find synonyms to search for. Search for alternative spellings of the word. Search for individual words rather than a phrase.
Too many results found	Use a more specific term. Search for a phrase rather than individual words. Narrow the search using Boolean "AND" if possible.

MEDLINE

Can't connect to site	Try another site. See MEDLINE section of http://www.medmatrix.org
Can't find any articles	Broaden your search by using a more general term. Search in a different field: subject, title word, keyword. Browse subject headings.
Too many articles	Use a more specific search term. Narrow your search to the current year. Narrow your search to a particular document type. Search by title word rather than any field.
Can't see an abstract for an article	Some articles don't have abstracts, such as letters to the editor.

EXERCISES

Each lettered exercise is independent.
(Links available at http://NewWindPub.com/workbook)

I. Guided Practice

A. MAKE A STARTUP DISK

WINDOWS 3.1

1. Double-click the Main program group.
2. Double-click File Manager.
3. In File Manager, click Disk, Make System Disk. Click Yes to "Are you sure..."
4. Click Start.

WINDOW 95

1. Put a blank 3½ inch floppy in the disk drive.
2. Click the Start button, then Settings, then Control Panel.
3. Double-click Add/Remove Programs.
4. Click the Startup Disk tab.
5. Click Create Disk.
6. Follow the instructions as it tells you to put a disk into the drive.

B. SCAN THE DISK FOR PHYSICAL PROBLEMS

Scanning can take 10-30 minutes, depending on the size of your hard drive. The program looks for physical defects. If it finds any, it will mark them so the computer doesn't use the defective areas in the future. Hard drives today are better than in the past, but scanning can be important for floppy disks.

WINDOWS 3.1
(REQUIRES DOS 6 OR HIGHER)

1. Exit Windows. (In Program Manager, click File, Exit. Click OK.)
2. When the screen is black and you see a command prompt (c:\...) type `scandisk`
3. Choose drive c:
4. The program will look through several different aspects of the drive.
5. If it finds a problem, you can usually choose "Fix it"

WINDOWS 95

1. Click the Start button, then Programs, Accessories, System Tools, Scan Disk.
2. Click Start.
3. ScanDisk will look through several different aspects of the drive.
4. If it finds a problem, you can usually choose "Fix it"

C. DEFRAGMENT THE HARD DRIVE

Defragmentation can take 10 minutes to several hours, depending on how fragmented your computer is and the speed of your processor.

WINDOWS 3.1 (REQUIRES DOS 6 OR HIGHER)

1. Exit Windows. (In Program Manager, click File, Exit. Click OK.)
2. When the screen is black and you see a command prompt (c:\...) type `defrag`
3. Choose drive c:
4. When defragmentation is done, tab to and press the Enter key.
5. Type win to return to Windows.

WINDOWS 95

1. Click the Start button, then Run...
2. Type `defrag` and click OK or press the Enter key.
3. At the window which says "Which drive do you want to defragment?" click OK.
4. Click Start.
5. When it is finished a window will appear "Do you wish to exit disk defragmenter?" Click OK.

D. RUN THE EMERGENCY RECOVERY UTILITY (ERU)

FROM THE CD

1. Insert your Windows 95 CD.
2. Start Explorer.
3. Click the drive letter for your CD drive.
4. Go to the Other/Misc/ERU subdirectory.
5. Double-click ERU.exe to start the program. Click Next.
6. Choose Other Directory. Click Next.
7. It will put the recovery files into c:\ERD. Click Next.
8. It shows you which files will be copied. Click Next.
9. If you need to run the recovery program, insert the system disk into the floppy drive.
10. At the a:\ prompt, type `c:`
11. At the c:\ prompt, type `cd eru`
12. At the c:\eru prompt, type `eru.exe`
13. This will start the recovery program.

FROM A DOWNLOADED COPY

1. Start Netscape or Explorer.
2. Go to http://www.microsoft.com/kb/articles/q139/4/37.htm
3. Download the zipped (compressed) eru.exe file from the link provided.
4. Use a compression program to expand the zip file.
5. If you don't have a compression program, see Appendix C.
6. Start eru.exe as above.

E. MAKE A BACKUP OF THE WINDOWS 95 REGISTRY

1. Insert your Windows 95 CD.
2. Start Explorer.
3. Click the drive letter for your CD drive.
4. Go to the Other/Misc/cfgback subdirectory.
5. Double-click Cfgback.exe
6. Click Continue through several screens.
7. At the text box "Selected Backup Name" type a descriptive name, for example the change you are about to make. E.g. `Before loading Netscape`
8. Click the Backup button.
9. You have now created a copy of the registry, which can be restored if the registry develops a problem later on.
10. To restore a backup of the registry, start the cfgback.exe program as above.
11. Select a backup from the list.
12. Click the Restore button.

F. EXPLORE MICROSOFT'S TROUBLESHOOTING AREA

This is an example of working through the Microsoft troubleshooting site to help solve a problem.

1. Start Netscape or Explorer.
2. Go to http://www.microsoft.com/support.
3. (Add a bookmark).
4. Click Troubleshooting Wizards.
5. Scroll down. Click the circular radio button next to "Windows 95: Solving problems starting..."
6. Click Next.
7. Click the radio button next to "My computer stops responding..."
8. Click Next.
9. Click the radio button next to "Yes, my computer boots to Safe mode."
10. Click Next.
11. You follow the screens in this way to determine a solution to your problem.

G. EXPLORE ZDNET'S TROUBLESHOOTING AREA

1. Start Netscape or Explorer.
2. Go to http://www.zdnet.com/hpc
3. (Add a bookmark).
4. Scroll down. Click Expert Advice.
5. Click Expert Answers for Windows 95
6. This is a forum hosted by ZDNet where you can post questions about Windows 95 and get answers. You must register (free) to post a question.

II. *Problem-Solving*

- Suppose that when you turn on your computer, you hear a humming noise as usual, but the screen doesn't show anything. What will you check first, second, third, etc.?
- A friend tells you "I can't connect to the Internet." What questions do you ask to figure out what she needs?
- It's five PM, you have a paper due tomorrow, and your computer won't start. What do you do?

III. *Thought and Discussion*

- Compare troubleshooting a computer to diagnosing an illness. How are they similar or different?
- Discuss experiences you have had with a computer help desk, then write up positive suggestions and send them to the manager of the help desk.
- Who is the most helpful nurse on your unit? What makes her helpful?

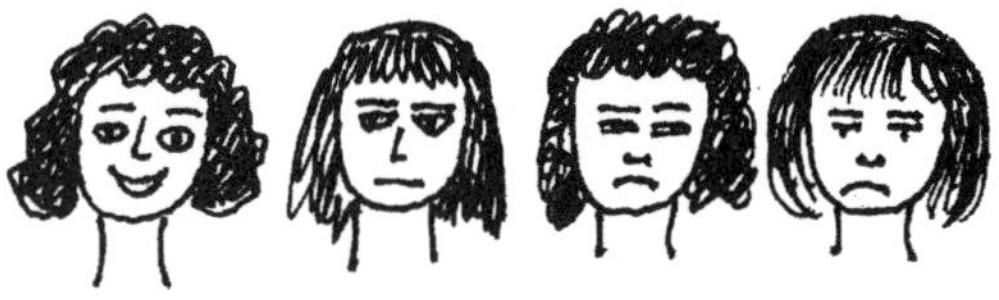

I give you four guesses!

- Think about new equipment and procedures you have had to learn, whether through classes, inservices, or hands-on training. How many of them have adequate manuals or other documentation? What is the best form for such documentation (pictures, help screens, step-by-step instructions)?

Readings from the Net

(Links available at http://NewWindPub.com/workbook)

Troubleshooting

BugNet	http://www.bugnet.com	Computer problems and their solutions. Free and registered areas.
HealthyPC.com	http://www.zdnet.com/hpc	Online advice, tips, troubleshooting.
Indiana University. Knowledge Base	http://sckb.ucssc.indiana.edu/kb	Well-constructed set of pages, links to other knowledge bases, clear answers.
Inquiry.com	http://www.inquiry.com	Search and find. Free registration.
MS Knowledge Base	http://www.microsoft.com/kb	Extensive and searchable.
News.com	http://www.news.com	For the latest that's happening.
TechWeb	http://www.techweb.com	A comprehensive technology site.
Viruses	http://www.cnet.com/Resources/Tech/Advisers/Virus	General description, tips, antivirus software.
Web Error Messages	http://www.cnet.com/Resources/Tech/Advisers/Error	What they are, and what to do about them.

Chapter 17: Creating Information

I have made this letter longer than usual, only because
I have not had the time to make it shorter.

Blaise Pascal, Lettres Provinciales, (1657)

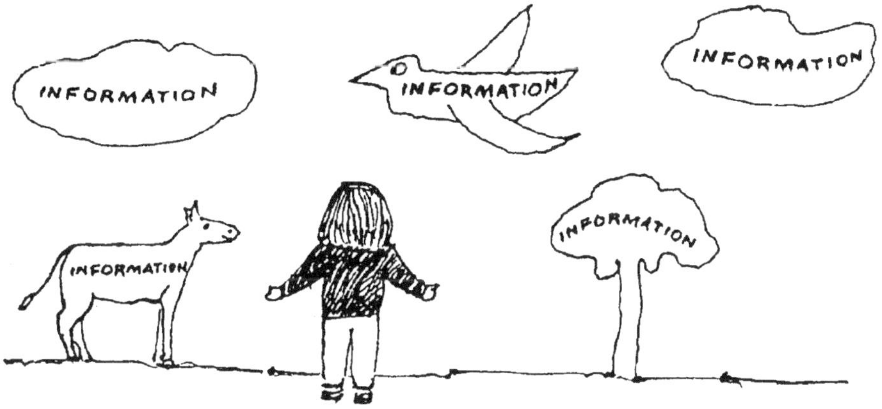

IN THIS CHAPTER

- cell
- chart
- clip art
- database
- desktop publishing
- field
- font
- form
- formula
- function
- header
- query
- spreadsheets
- suite
- template
- thesaurus
- word processing

We are all creators: every day is an adventure in discussion, thought, writing. As a healthcare professional you can use information tools for more effective research, communication, and teaching. What is more, information will soon be integrated in a way that was unthinkable even a few years ago. After composing a report it will be possible to publish it on the Internet, share it in a whiteboard conference, or illustrate it with graphics from a worldwide collection of images.

First, however, you must become familiar with basic concepts and programs. This chapter and the exercises which follow will do that. The basics of any program can be learned in a few hours, but producing a finished work takes time. "I don't know that there are any short cuts to doing a good job." (Sandra Day O'Conner) More than any other kind of work, information follows the 80/20 rule: the last 20% (usually fine details) takes as much time as the first 80%. Be prepared for that. Because the tools are available, more of us are called upon to create a newsletter, slide show, database, Web presentation. Oh—remember to save documents often, or that fine brainwork might become bits down the digital drain if the power goes out.

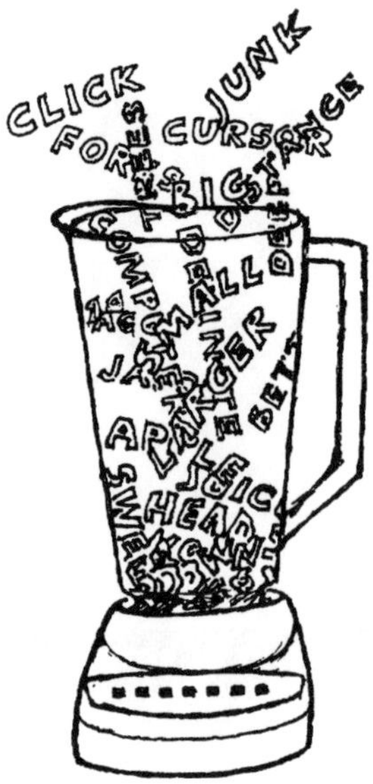

Word Processing

Common programs: MS Word, Word Perfect, PageMaker

Writing is an art we all share, and with a little attention, one that gives pleasure to both author and reader. Virginia Woolf says, "How delightful to feel [a sentence] form and curve under my fingers!" The purpose of a word processor, like an electric typewriter, is to create written documents, and probably the most important aspect of a word processor is the ability to save your document and work on it later.

After you start most word processing programs, you can begin typing immediately.

To move back to a section you have typed, click in that section with the mouse. This positions the cursor. Now you can use the delete or backspace keys to erase, or you can type new words in the middle of a sentence.

Selecting Text

To change the look of the words you have typed, you must first select them. Click and hold the mouse button next to a sentence and drag across the sentence. This highlights the words. Release the mouse button. Move the pointer up to the button bar and click the button which has the letter ***B*** on it. Your sentence will now be bold. The same approach works for underlining, italics, size of text, centering, even the color of the text.

If you don't know what the buttons in a program are for, position the mouse pointer over one for a few seconds. You do not need to click. A box will appear with the name or description for that button.

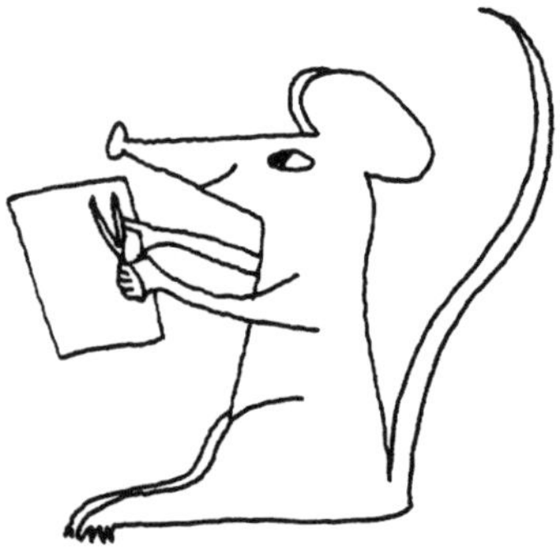

Moving Text: Cut, Copy, Paste

You can move text in two ways. One is by first selecting the text, then using drag and drop to move it to a new location. With the second method, you select the text, then use the Edit, Cut menu choice. The text will disappear. Click the mouse to position the cursor where you want the text to go, then click Edit, Paste. (In Windows 95, the cut and paste commands pop up when you right-click after selecting text. Try it.)

> *Undo*
>
> A menu function that can reverse mistakes.

Undo

The Edit menu often includes an Undo item, which reverses the last action you took. This is invaluable, especially in the beginning when you don't know what went wrong.

Tables

A table lets you present structured information in a manner that is easy to see and understand. This is a table with two rows and four columns:

Columns

You can format your text so it flows in two or more columns, like a newspaper or magazine. This is often easier to read, and gives you extra space to put pictures, headlines, quotes, and other items.

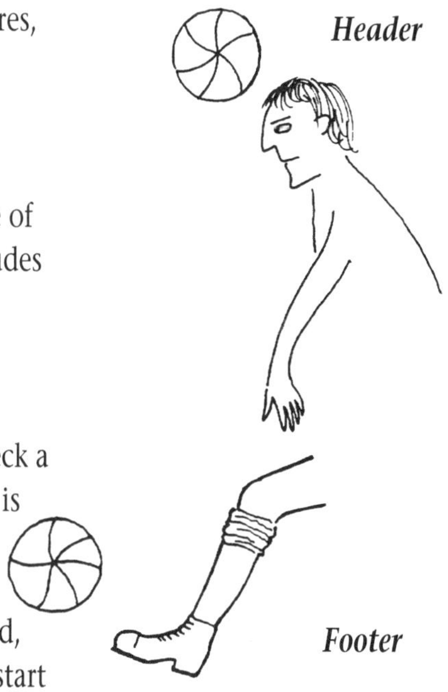

Headers and Footers

A header is something that appears at the top of every page, such as the title of the document. A footer appears at the bottom of every page, and often includes the page number.

Spelling Checker

Most programs will now check the spelling of your words. MS Word will check a document as you type, and put a jagged line underneath any word it thinks is misspelled. You can then right-click the word to see a suggested spelling.

You can also have the document checked for spelling as a whole. In MS Word, click the Tools, Spelling menu. A window will pop up and the program will start to look at your document. It will stop at any word not found in its dictionary, and suggest alternatives. You can choose to ignore the suggested alternatives, type in a correction, or insert the correct spelling. In MS Word you can also right-click a word to see a suggested spelling.

Even though a program can check for spelling, it is still a good idea to proof your writing. Spell checkers will miss some errors, such as typing "is" instead of "it."

Thesaurus

A thesaurus is a list of synonyms and antonyms. In MS Word, select a word, then click the Tools, Thesaurus menu. A window will pop up with synonyms. Double-click any word to see synonyms for the new word. In this way you can look through a large number of related words very quickly. Click the Replace button to substitute a synonym for your original word.

Template

A preset format, such as for a publication.

Newsletters, Brochures, Memos

Word processors have preformatted templates which you can use to create a newsletter, brochure, memo, resume, or other specific kind of publication. The layout of the columns, titles, page numbering, even a table of contents is already done. All you have to do is fill in the words.

An entire document can be saved as a template, so that the format (title, paragraphs, etc.) can be used again and again. This can help with standard forms, reports, or memos.

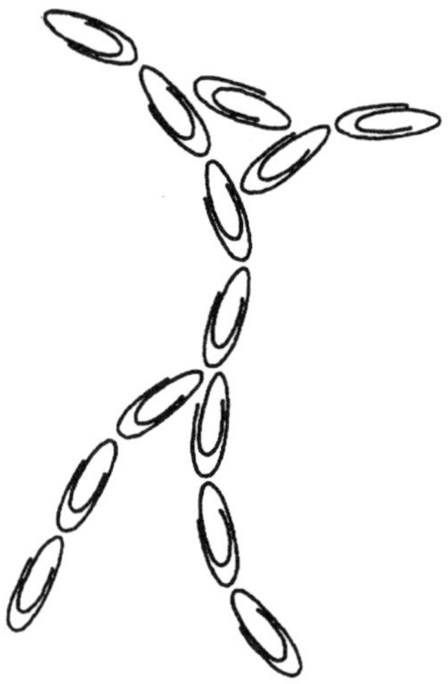

Clip Art

Most programs now come with a few dozen built-in images that you can insert into a document. In addition, you can buy libraries of several thousand digital images for $30-50 to use in publications. In MS Word, click Insert, Picture to try this function.

Styles

If you are writing a long and complex document you can set up special styles for repeated elements such as chapter titles, subheadings, bibliography entries, footnotes, or Internet addresses. Then when you want to change the format (size of the text, bold, italic) of these items, you simply change the style, and all the entries will change.

Indexing

You can build an automatic index for the back of a book or article. In MS Word, start at the beginning of the document. Select a word, then use Insert, Index. On the Index tab of the window that pops up, click Mark Entry. Repeat for the other words you want in your index. At the end, position the cursor where you want the index, then click Insert, Index.

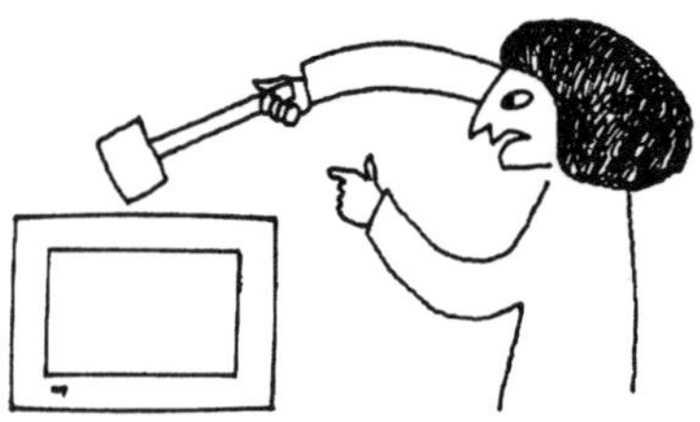

Automatic Save

In the Tools, Options, Save menu of MS Word, you can specify how often the program will automatically save your document. Set this to five or ten minutes. I once sat next to a clinical specialist who had worked for eight hours on a report, when suddenly the power went off for a fraction of a second. The computer shut down, and all her work was lost. Better to save often than beat a defenseless machine in a fit of rage.

Much more...

A word processor can do much more: cross-references, date and time, page numbering, bulleted and numbered lists, word counts, annotations by reviewers, special symbols (@ © ¶ ™). These may seem like small potatoes compared to the ideas and facts in a document, but every detail, correctly placed, adds to the whole.

Spreadsheet

Common programs: Excel, Lotus123

> *Cell*
>
> One of the small boxes in a spreadsheet.

A spreadsheet uses an arrangement of rows and columns to perform automatic calculations. On the screen it looks like one big table:

	A	*B*	*C*	*D*	*E*	*F*	*G*	*H*
1								
2		15						
3		20						
4		10						
5		15						
6		*60*						
7								

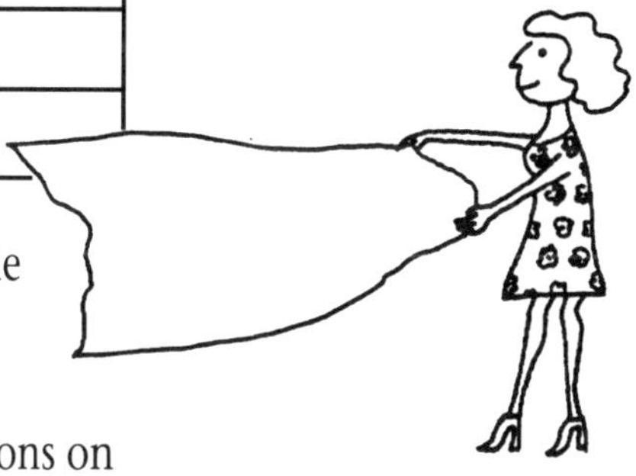

Each box, or cell, in a spreadsheet has an address such as A1, B1, A2, B2. The numbers in the spreadsheet above are in cells B2 through B7.

Within each cell an algebraic formula can be placed which will do calculations on the numbers from other cells and display the result. For example, the formula in cell B6 is (B2+B3+B4+B5).

A spreadsheet also includes a library of ready-to-use formulas, called functions, which can apply to a group of numbers. For example, in cell B7 is the formula "PROD (B2:B6)", which multiplies these numbers and gives the product.

When a number is changed in any cell, the formulas recalculate automatically.

The numbers and results can be automatically graphed. Spreadsheets can be used to track costs, create staffing sheets, or conduct research.

Database

Common programs: Access, Paradox, Dbase, FoxPro

A database program keeps track of information. An addressbook is a simple database with name, address, and telephone number for people. The patient database in a hospital or clinic is simply an expanded addressbook, with fields for unit number, date of birth, number of admissions, and so on.

The information in a database is stored in a table; this looks much like a spreadsheet:

Unit Number	*First*	*Last*	*Age*	*Sex*	*Diagnosis*
4445556	Peter	Pickle	2	M	croup
6665444	Jane	Juniper	10	F	tinnitus
5554666	Cracker	Jack	15	M	fever
1111111	Dave	Dolittle	9	M	lassitude

Each column in a database is called a field; a field can hold a number, text, graphic, sound, or video. All the information on one person is called a record.

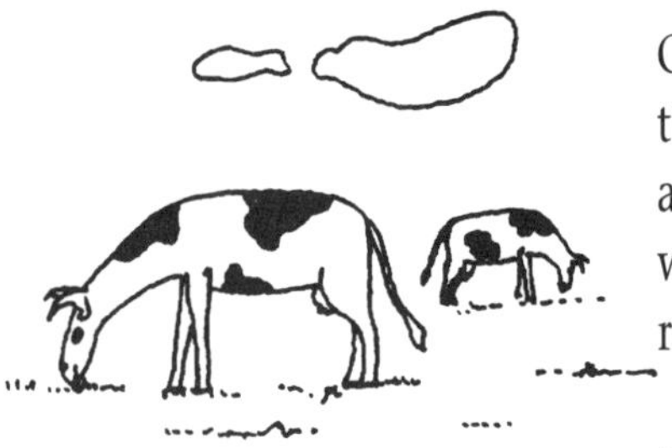

Field of cows

Once information has been entered into a database, there are a number of things that can be done with it. The information can be sorted by any of the fields, or an automatic question (query) can be set up. For example, "Show me all the records where a patient is over ten years old and had a diagnosis of fever." A automatic report can be generated that prints out the entire table, or the results of a query.

Relational databases were invented in 1970 by E. F. Codd. Visualize a three-dimensional checkers board, and you have a good idea of a relational database: a series of related tables. A business might set up a customer table, an invoice table, and an inventory table, then link them all together as one relational database. A customer can then be related to several invoices, or one invoice related to several items of inventory.

Record

All the information on one item in a database.

Databases and the Web

A database can be created with a personal computer, and then linked to a Web page. A standard language has been developed, called SQL (Structured Query Language) that programmers use to put information into or retrieve it from a database. A similar standard, based on SQL, is called ODBC (Open Database Connect). SQL and OBDC are used by Web programmers for accessing database information, and for creating dynamic Web pages which are created immediately before they are displayed.

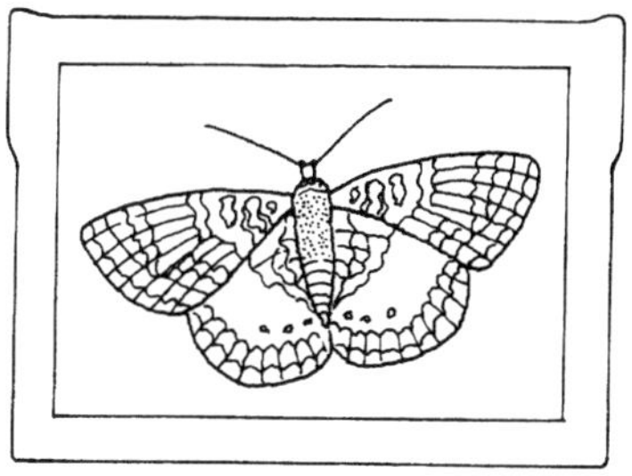

Graphic Presentation

Common programs: PowerPoint, Harvard Graphics.

A graphic presentation program creates a series of screens (slides) for use in a teaching presentation. These are relatively easy programs to learn and use.

First you should decide upon the overall design for the slide show. The program has a number of templates with different styles and colors. Once you choose this master template, those borders and colors will appear automatically on each slide.

For each slide you determine the overall type of information: a title, a bulleted list, a pie chart, etc. Then enter the information, or insert it from another program. (You can import a spreadsheet, database, graphic, text, or other information directly into your presentation. Or you can use the copy and paste functions described in the word processing section above.)

With these tools at your fingertips, you can do much more than was possible even a few years ago. We are all capable of greatness—or at least a newsletter! On a related point Stephen Jay Gould wrote, "Giants have not ceded to mere mortals, rather the boundaries...have been restricted and the edges smoothed."

EXERCISES

Each lettered exercise is independent.
(Links available at http://NewWindPub.com/workbook)

I. Guided Practice

A. BASIC WORD PROCESSING

WRITE (WINDOWS 3.1) AND WORDPAD WINDOWS 95

MS Write is a small word processing program that comes with Windows 3.1. WordPad is the Windows 95 version. These are excellent programs to learn word processing because they come with the computer and are uncomplicated. Below you will learn basic functions that are available in most word processing programs. Neither program has advanced functions such as spell checking or tables.

START THE PROGRAM

1. (Windows 3.1) Double-click the Accessories program group to open it.
2. Double-click the icon above the word Write. (Windows 95) Click the Start button, then Programs, Accessories, then WordPad.
3. (Or click Start, Run. Type `wordpad` and press the Enter key.)

EXPAND THE WINDOW AND FONT

1. Double-click the title bar (to the right of the word "Write - Untitled" (Windows 95: "WordPad") to expand the window to full-screen.
2. Click the Character, Enlarge Font menu. (Windows 95: click the triangle next to the number 10. Click 12 to enlarge the default font size.

TYPE SOME TEXT

1. Type the following stanza from a song by Garrison Keillor. Press the Enter key after each line.

```
A cat can lie flat on its back
And never be ambitious;
Where the grass is sweet
Beneath your feet,
And the houseplants are delicious.
```

MOVE TEXT

1. Click to the right of the first line.
2. Press the Enter key to create a blank line.
3. Click to the right of the last line and drag the pointer across the entire line until it is highlighted.
4. Click the Edit, Cut menu. The line should disappear.
5. Click once in the blank line.
6. Click Edit, Paste. The line should reappear in the new spot.

CHANGE TEXT CHARACTERISTICS

1. Click to the right of the last line and drag the pointer across the entire line until it is highlighted.
2. Click the Character, Bold menu. Then click Character, Italic menu. (Windows 95: Click the B and I on the button bar.)
3. The line should now be bold and italic.
4. Click the Paragraph, Center menu. (Windows 95: Format, Paragraph. At the bottom of the window, click the word Left and choose Center instead.)
5. Click OK. The line should now be centered on the page.

AUTOMATIC REPLACE

1. Click Find, Replace menu. (Windows 95: Edit, Replace.)
2. In the Find What box, type `stops`
3. In the Replace With box, type `sits`
4. Click the Replace button, then Replace All, then Close. (Windows 95: Click the Replace All button. Click OK, then Close.)
5. The word "stops" has been replaced by the word "sits."

BULLETED LIST

(Only in Wordpad - Windows 95)

1. Click at the beginning of the poem.
2. Drag to the end of the third line to highlight all three lines.
3. Click Format, Bullet Style.
4. Each line now has a bullet in front of it.

UNDO

1. (Windows 3.1) Catch up with the last exercise: Click at the beginning of the poem. Drag to the end of the third line to highlight all three lines.
2. Click Paragraph, Center menu. (Windows 95: Click Format, Paragraph. Click the word Left and choose Center.)
3. Click anywhere on the page.
4. To undo the last action, click Edit, Undo.

5. The three lines should move to the left. Undo lets you reverse the last action. In some programs you can keep clicking Undo to move back through a series of actions.

SAVE THE DOCUMENT

1. Click the File, Save menu.
2. Type `stuff.wri` (Windows 95: `stuff.doc`)
3. Click the Save button or press the Enter key.
4. Your document is now saved.
5. Click File, Exit to close the program.

OPEN A FILE FROM THE DISK

1. Start the program as above.
2. Click the File menu.
3. Note that because your document was open recently, it appears in a list at the bottom. You can click this to open it. But don't.
4. Click Open.
5. If you don't see your file, use the scroll bar at the bottom of the Open window to look for it.
6. Click the file named stuff.wri or stuff.doc, then click Open or press the Enter key.
7. Your file should appear.

LOOK AT A PREVIEW OF THE FILE FOR PRINTING
(Only in WordPad - Windows 95)

1. Click the File, Print Preview menu.
2. Click Zoom In to enlarge the image.
3. Click Zoom Out to shrink it again.
4. Click Close to return to the editing screen.

CHANGE THE VIEW OF THE PROGRAM ONSCREEN
(Only in WordPad - Windows 95)

1. Click the View menu.
2. Click Format Bar.
3. The toolbar with buttons for bold, italic, etc. will disappear.
4. Click View, Format Bar again to reverse the change.

II. Problem-Solving

- Create a newsletter with your word processor using a preformatted style or template.
- Write a paragraph with your word processor. Then spend fifteen minutes with the thesaurus function finding alternative words. Compare the two paragraphs. Any improvement?

Thought and Discussion

- Bring a copy of *Wired Magazine*, *PC Magazine*, and a nursing journal to class. Discuss the layout of each in terms of usefulness, ease of reading, and appeal.
- Present a table of numbers as a table, a graph, and a narrative description. Then compare the usefulness of each type of presentation.
- Loren Eiseley, a noted writer and paleontologist, says that "the attempt to leap forward into the future [is] a phenomenon of our turbulent era." Are the information tools mentioned in this chapter really necessary for your work?

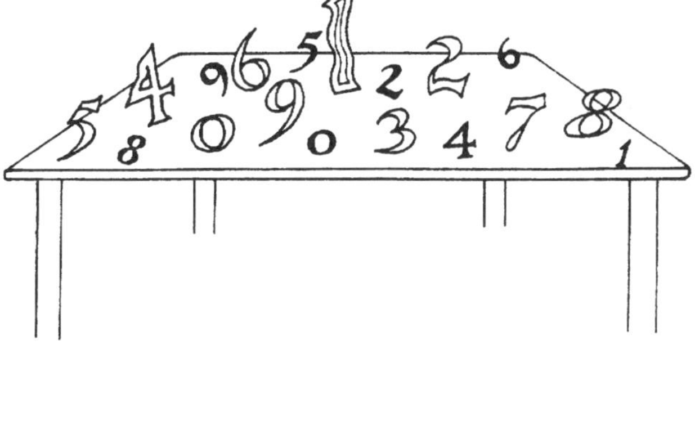

Chapter 18: New Career Choices

Life is either a daring adventure or it is nothing.
Helen Keller

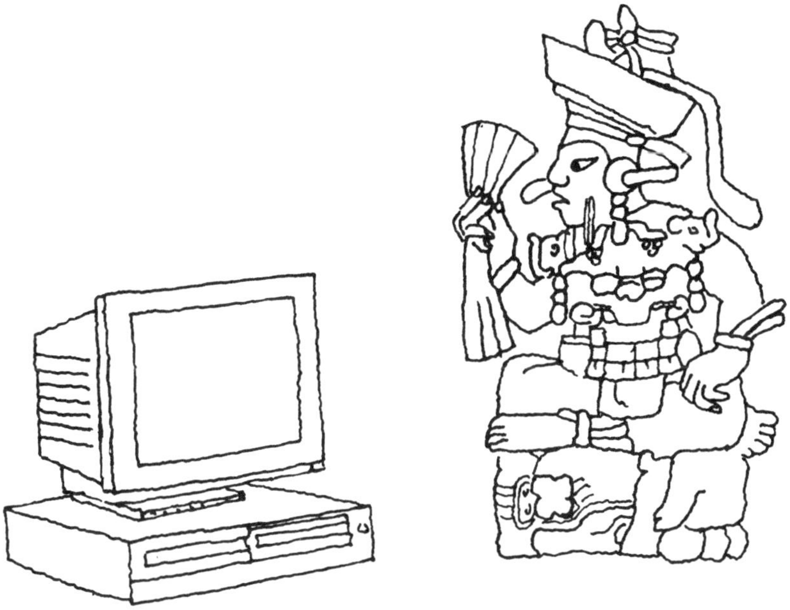

IN THIS CHAPTER

clinical education
clinical information system
database development
intranet
journal club
networking
patient education
research
Web publishing
Web team

No matter what happens, two fields are going to need people in the next century: health care and computers. Expertise in either field will mean a job; expertise in both means you can create your own position. You don't need to keep your nose to the grindstone, just your ear to the ground, because that's not an earthquake, it's the Net shaking up our future history. And if you think that you don't have anything to contribute, think again: your hospital information department may not have the foggiest idea what clinical professionals do, or what they need.

Clinical Information System

Does your hospital have a computer system that integrates orders, radiology images, admission/discharge/transfer (ADT) data, monitors, narrative charting, laboratory results, outpatient visits, flow sheets, drip rates, medications, and problem lists? If not, chances are good that the board of directors is actively researching such a system. Called clinical information systems, electronic medical records, or computerized patient records, they can do all of the above; in the near future they will also include email, Web links to MEDLINE, teaching handouts, exchange of data with other institutions, telemedicine for distant consults, and more.

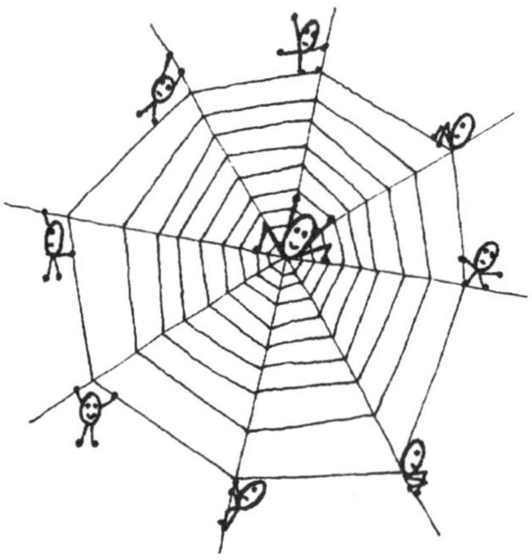

Teamwork is essential for the planning, installation and maintenance of a clinical information system, with the most important contribution coming from clinical personnel in medicine, nursing, respiratory care, etc. Engineers and programmers can get the system up and running, but clinicians are needed to ensure that the screens have the right information, in a format that clinicians can work with.

Web Team

Most hospitals and health care institutions now have some sort of Web site, but the vast majority are little more than a few pages of public relations. Five or ten years from now most institutional documents (patient teaching handouts, formularies, policies) and much else will be found on intranets. Somebody will have to put them there.

> *intranet*
>
> A network designed to exchange information within an organization using TCP/IP.

In recent years, creating Web documents required a person to learn hypertext markup language (HTML). At that time the term "Webmaster" referred to the person who set up the Web server, created the site, wrote most of the materials, edited pages for other people, and sharpened the pencils. Today many companies are realizing that it takes a team of people to create and maintain a Web site, just as it takes a team to produce a newsletter or television show.

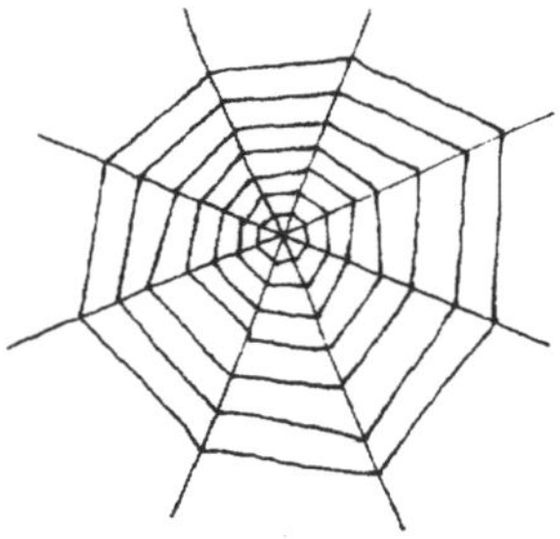

A good healthcare Web team should include an editor to oversee the whole project, a programmer to maintain the Web server and related programs, several specialists to organize the content, and an assistant to convert and format documents. A health professional is an asset in any of these positions, except perhaps for technical programming.

In addition to this team, it is useful to have a committee of representatives from different departments: administration, OR, ER, outpatient. Email and other methods make it easy to collaborate on individual projects.

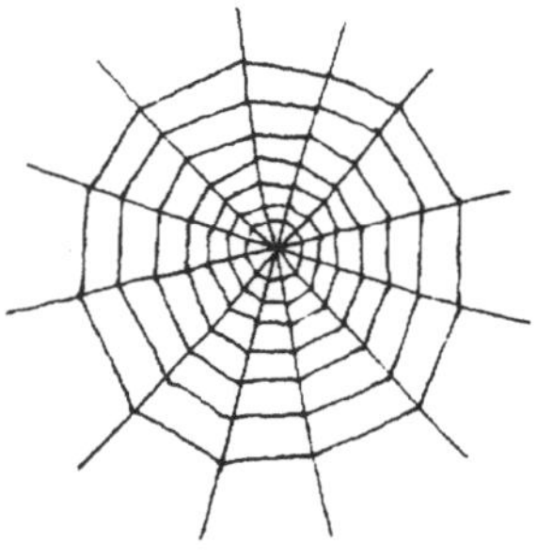

Publishing on the Web

From now on most programs will have the capacity to convert documents to Web (HTML) format. If you have the latest version of any major word processor, you can do this easily. But if you want to manage an entire Web site, rather than just create individual pages, you will need to learn one of the more complete site-management tools such as Claris HomePage, Macromedia Designer, Microsoft FrontPage, Adobe PageMill, or Quarterdeck WebAuthor.

Keep in mind that HTML and the Web are changing. You will need to keep up with new programs, formats, and standards as they emerge.

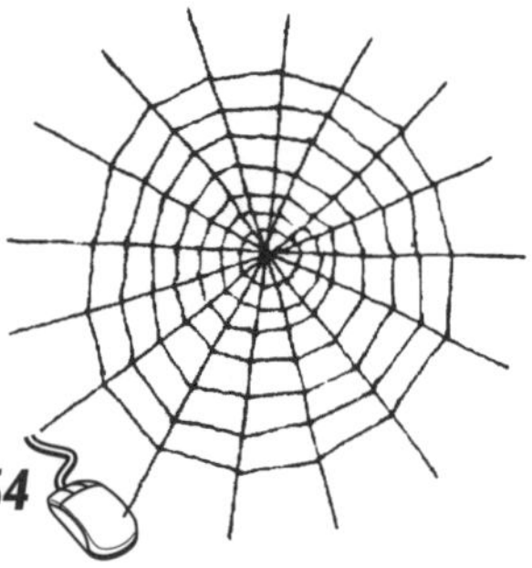

Clinical Medical and Nursing Education

Traditionally, clinical educators have a background in patient care, and if they are lucky, some experience with education. What most of them don't have is an understanding of computer and information tools. Education departments today have libraries for course material, handouts, recordings, and videos. They need people to convert these to digital format, create online courses ("computer-based training," CBT), online registration, interactive classes, and continuing education.

Multimedia refers to anything more than text on a computer screen, such as sound, video, animation, or three-dimensional graphics. Macromedia Director and Authorware are two popular programs for creating multimedia presentations on the Web, but many programs can produce similar results.

Business Process Reengineering

This is a big, ugly phrase for a simple concept: streamlining. Most activities involve separate steps (for example: write an order, send it to pharmacy, deliver the drug to the unit, get the drug from the cart, prepare the drug, give it to the patient). Any process can be improved, and the Web is now available to help. Look at what Federal Express, United Parcel Service, or Amazon.com have done with the Web. Imagine what you could do—then do it!

Patient Education

There are many opportunities here, especially with the ongoing trend towards home care and health maintenance organizations. Education is central to preventive medicine and home care. What is managed care but the management of information? As more people get access to computers, patient education can be vastly expanded, courses can be tailored to specific groups, and the effect of education can be tracked automatically.

Within hospitals, personal computers can be used in a number of innovative ways for patient education. The Sacramento Public Library has had a computer-based kiosk for the past few years which describes the library collection. Imagine having an interactive computer station that patients could use to watch videos, get handouts, search for information on diseases—all while sitting in the waiting room or even the exam room.

Database Development

Personal computers have the speed and storage capacity to work with large databases, and programs are available (such as dBase or MS Access) that non-programmers can learn. Institutions need health care professionals who can design, build, and maintain databases.

Every department or work area can benefit from an organized (database) approach to the collection and analysis of information. A few examples are clinical research, inventory tracking, analysis of procedures, or staffing.

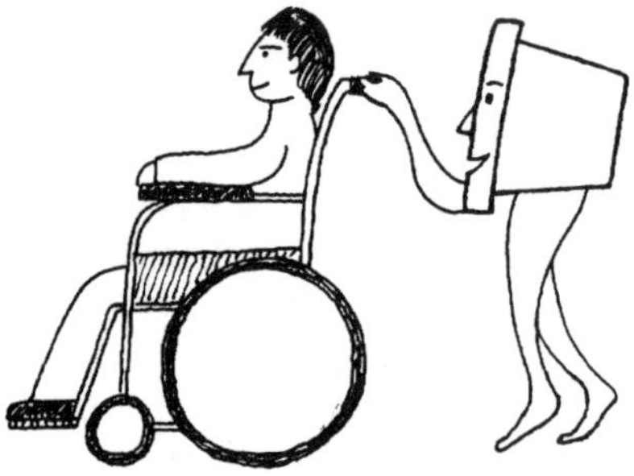

The Disabled

In the past, personal computers were either too expensive or too limited to be of much use to the disabled. But this is changing. In the next few years speech recognition will become accessible to everyone: we will be able to run a computer by talking rather than typing. Healthcare providers are needed to develop these technologies and work with those who will use them. "Service is what life is all about," says Marion Wright Edelman, founder of the Children's Defense Fund.

Whiteboard

A program that lets people who are in different locations simultaneously see text or pictures.

Networking With Professionals

Although email and mailing lists have been crucial for electronic collaboration, a new generation of tools are becoming available, such as Web sites, whiteboards, videoconferences, and telemedicine. Most professionals don't understand these very well, if at all. If you can bring people together and you understand how to use the Internet, you will be in high demand. Who better to do this than nurses? Lewis Thomas, MD makes a familiar observation in *The Youngest Science*: "My discovery, as a patient first on the medical service and later in surgery, is that the institution is held together, *glued* together...by the nurses and by nobody else." The word for the next decade is "collaboration."

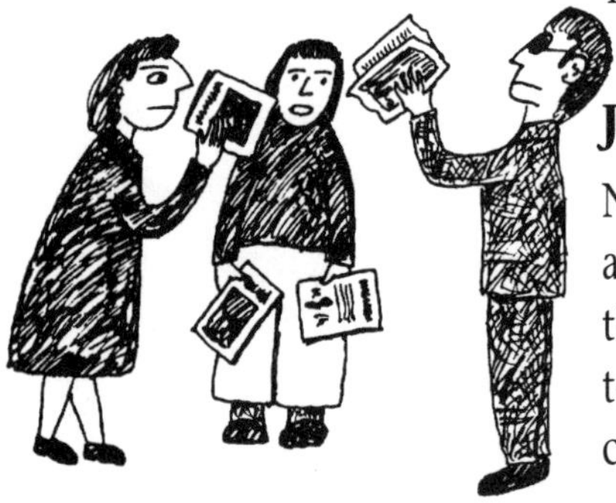

Journal Club

Now that MEDLINE is on the Internet, and as more publishers put up full-text articles, it is easier than ever to research new medical procedures and to share them with peers. A journal club traditionally picks an article to read, then gathers to discuss it. Today you can use a Web site or email list to conduct discussions, create links to abstracts or full-text articles, even contact authors.

Research

Every week I get informal requests from friends and coworkers to do research for them on the Internet. They have Internet access and understand a little about email and the Web, but are not very skilled at finding a particular piece of information quickly.

Take a survey of students or professionals: ask how many are able to sit down at a computer with Internet access and pull up guidelines, clinical trials, patient handouts, clinical education courses, drug references, bibliographic citations? If you have worked through this book from the beginning, you can probably arrange a series of bookmarks to do just that in no time at all. You may discover, after working through this book, that you are in high demand.

Imminent Death of the Net Predicted!

Don't believe all you read about the Internet: it's here to stay, and a lot of good is coming from it. Dystopias are out of fashion. In the new information-rich world of the Internet we need health professionals who are familiar with these vast resources. However, not all of us will learn at the same pace—or need to. Olaf Stapledon described our situation well: "Long before the human spirit awoke to clear cognizance of the world and itself, it sometimes stirred in its sleep, opened bewildered eyes, and slept again."

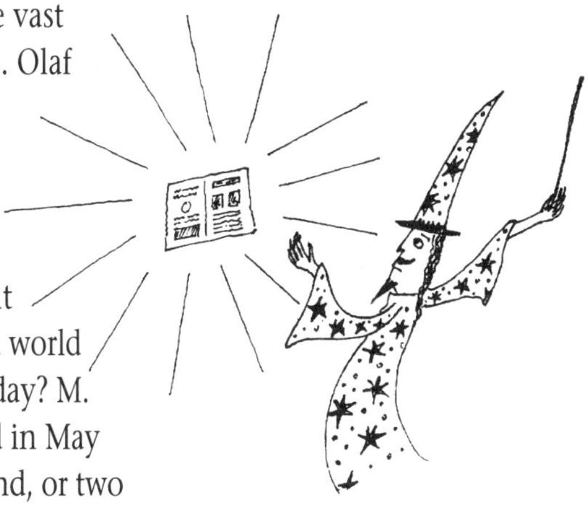

Much of the world is asleep to the potential of the Internet, but slowly it is awakening. Internet II is coming, schools are getting wired, many third world countries are investing in computer systems. Should you wait, or start today? M. Stuart Lynn, Associate Vice President for the University of California, said in May 1997: "When's the future? Is it one hundred years from now, one thousand, or two years?" For healthcare professionals the Internet may be a swim in the ocean of knowledge, or a link to the the extended community of healthcare professionals, or a tool for improving the health of millions. I hope this book has helped, and that you use it to join the awakening world-mind that is the Internet. Look me up when you get there.

EXERCISES

(Links available at http://NewWindPub.com/workbook)

II. Problem-Solving

- Interview the computer support person for your school or hospital, then present a ten-minute description of the computer systems.

III. Thought and Discussion

- Who is an "information professional"?
- How much of the work in nursing and medicine deals with information, as compared to physical, hands-on care?
- How much of the work in nursing and medicine involves coordination which could be streamlined through the availability of immediate information, e.g., lab reports, patient schedules, bed assignments?
- Imagine a state-of-the-art hospital twenty-five years in the future. What will the nursing information managers be doing?

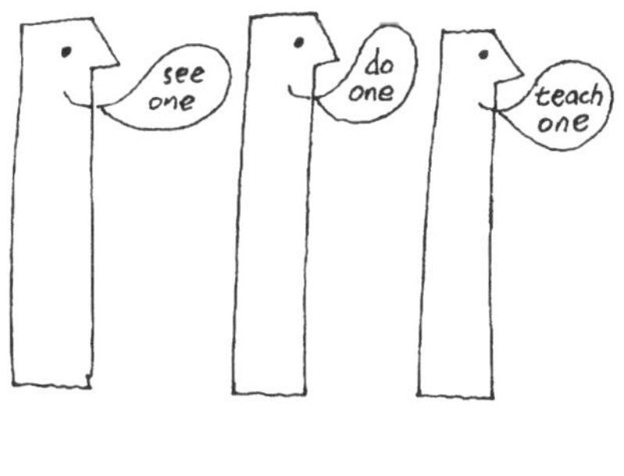

Readings from the Net

(Links available at http://NewWindPub.com/workbook)

Internet, Informatics, and Health Care

Computers and Medicine	http://www.acponline.org/journals/news/compmed.htm	Fifty full-text articles from the ACP Observer, January 1995-present.
Healthcare Informatics	http://www.mcis.duke.edu/standards/guide.htm	Everything about Informatics: standards, organizations, coding, specialty info.
Health Data Management	http://hdm.fgray.com	For CEO's. Major issues discussed.
Internet and Health Care	http://www.ey.com/health/internethc.htm	Brief into. Full document is 1.8 MB, pdf
WWW and the Electronic Medical Record	http://www.med.virginia.edu/~wmd4n/WWWTalk/WWW-outline.html	Notes from a talk given Nov. 1994 by Dr. William Detmer.

Web publishing

How to Publish Your Web Site	http://www.cnet.com/Content/Features/Howto/Publish	Friendly introduction. Links to advanced topics, program reviews.
Web Authoring	http://www.pcmag.com/iu/author/wysiwyg/_wysiwyg.htm	Reviews and download links for all the major programs.

Employment Directories

ABC Med. Computing	http://www.bmj.com/bmj/abcmc/abcmc.htm	An abridged version of their book.
AJN Career Guide	http://www.ajn.org	Guide and essays.
America's Job Bank	http://www.ajb.dni.us	Job listings.
Excite Job page	http://www.excite.com/xdr/Business/Jobs	Plenty of sites and reviews.
Health Careers Online	http://www.healthcareers-online.com	Job listings in health care.
Health Search USA	http://www.healthsearchusa.com	Physician recruitment.
JobWeb	http://www.jobweb.org	Good for recent graduates.
Medical Matrix job page	http://www.medmatrix.org/SPages/Employment.stm	Links to and reviews of several dozen medical employment sites.
The Monster Board	http://www.monster.com	National and international.
Nursing Informatics	http://www.ajn.org/other/ncnr/report/title.html	May 1993 report. Dense, abstract.
The Riley Guide	http://www.jobtrak.com/jobguide	Excellent general starting page.
TechWeb career page	http://www.techweb.com/careers/careers.html	Good resource for technical jobs.

A MEDICAL INTERNET BOOKS

1997 Guide to Health Care Resources on the Internet	Hoben, 1997
Computers in Clinical Practice	Osheroff, 1995
Health Net	Ryer, 1997
Health on the Internet	Anthony, 1996
The Internet for Nurses and Allied Health Professionals	Edwards, 1997
The Internet for Physicians	Smith, 1997
Internet Guide for the Health Professional, 2nd Ed.	Hogarth & Hutchinson, 1996
Internet pour les Médecins, 2me	Cassagne, 1997
Internet Workbook for Health Professionals	Hutchinson, 1997
Medical Information on the Internet	Kiley, 1996
Medicine and the Internet	Pareras, 1996
Medicine and the Internet: Introducing Online Resources and Terminology	McKenzie, 1996
Nurses' Guide to the Internet	Nicoll, 1997
The Online Guide to Healthcare Management & Medicine	Goldstein & Flory, 1997
Physicians' Guide to the Internet	Hancock, 1996
Pocket Guide to the Medical Internet	Hutchinson, 1997

B List of Guided Exercises

Chapter 1: No Experience Necessary

Forward, Back, Home buttons
Go menu
Type an address (Location bar)
Type an address (File menu)
Netscape home page
Search for a word (Find function)
Right-click (Forward, Back)
Add a bookmark

Chapter 2: Windows and Your Computer

Open a program group
Start a program
Enlarge to full screen
Save a document
Close a program
Open a document
Print a document
Alt-Tab switching
Move files
Drag and drop files
Rename a file
Copy a file from floppy to hard drive
Find a file
Delete a file
Recover a deleted file (Windows 95)
Online help (Windows 95)

Chapter 3: Netscape Navigator and Microsoft Explorer

Email a Web page
Copy a Web page
Add a bookmark to a page
Save a page as a file
Determine length of a Web page for printing

Chapter 4: Anatomy of a Website

Button bar, frames
Mailto link
Forum
Web chat
Imagemaps and thumbnails
Banners & MEDLINE

Chapter 5: Electronic Mail

Set up Eudora or Nedscape to receive and send mail
Send a message
Add a name to the addressbook
Use an email alias
Send a Cc with a message
Send an attached file
Check for new messages
Open an attachment
Delete a message
Reply to a message
Create a mailbox folder
Transfer a message to a folder

Chapter 6: Bookmarks

Save a bookmark
Create a bookmark folder
File a bookmark (Netscape 4)
Drag a bookmark
Put a folder within a folder
Rename a bookmark
Right-click to create a bookmark
Right-click to create a shortcut

Chapter 7: Online Directories

Medical Matrix
MedMark
MedWeb
Health section of Excite
Specialty directory (nursing)

Chapter 8: Searching

Excite
Medical World
CliniWeb
Browse MeSH categories
Medis

Health on the Net
AltaVista
Metacrawler

Chapter 9: MEDLINE and CINAHL

MEDLINE:
Search NLM's Web site
Abstracts
Related articles
Help
Advanced Search
Fields
Listing terms
Add terms to a search
Search for a phrase
Publication types
Modify the search
Search for a truncated word

CINAHL:
Run a search
View short form
Search for a journal
Limit to a type of article
Save results to a file
Save the search strategy
Search the permuted index
Look at subheadings

Chapter 10: Patient Education

HealthFinder
National Health Information Center
Toll-free numbers
MedHelp
Medical Glossary
HealthAnswers

Chapter 11: Medical Journals and News

Cable News Network health site
Newspage
Linked news stories
Find a journal
Nursing article search
AMA site

Chapter 12: Medical Sites

(none)

Chapter 13: Ethics, Law, Responsibility

(none)

Chapter 14: Mailing Lists, Discussion Groups

Open a newsgroup
Post a message to a group

Chapter 15: Managing Time and Information

(none)

Chapter 16: Troubleshooting

Make a startup disk
Scan the hard drive
Defragment the hard drive
Run the Emergency Recovery Utility (Windows 95)
Backup the Registry (Windows 95)
Explore Microsoft's troubleshooting area
Explore ZDNet's troubleshooting area

Chapter 17: Creating Information

Change font size
Cut and paste text
Change text characteristics
Find and replace text
Bulleted list
Undo
Save a document
Open a file from the disk
Print preview
Show Toolbar

Chapter 18: New Career Choices

(none)

Software on the Internet

(Links available at http://
NewWindPub.com/workbook)

Software Libraries

Coast to Coast	http://www.coast.net/SimTel
Filez	http://www.filez.com
Oakland	http://oak.oakland.edu
Shareware	http://shareware.com
Softseek	http://www.softseek.com
TUCOWS	http://tucows.hunterlink.net.au

Browsers, email, ftp, winsock

Calaveras	http://www.caltel.com/wares.html
Preferred	http://www.preferred.com

Email

Eudora	http://www.qualcomm.com
Pronto	http://www.commtouch.com
Pegasus	http://www.pegasus.usa.com/welcome.htm

Document Viewers

Acrobat	http://www.adobe.com
Envoy	http://www.twcorp.com

Anti-Virus

McAfee	http://www.mcafee.com
Norton	http://www.norton.com
ViruSafe	http://www.eliashim.com

Compression

PKZip	http://www.pkware.com
Stuffit for Windows	http://www.aladdinsys.com

Animation and Multimedia

Shockwave	http://www.macromedia.com/shockwave

Audio and Music

RealAudio	http://www.realaudio.com
TrueSpeech	http://www.dspg.com
Liquid Music Player	http://www.liquidaudio.com
MidiPlug	http://www.ysba.com/midplug_index.html

Video

VDOLive Player	http://www.vdolive.com
VivoActive	http://www.vivo.com
InterVU Player	http://www.interu.com
Cuseeme	http://www.cu-seeme.com
Quicktime	http://quicktime.apple.com

Virtual Reality

VRML Repository	http://www.sdsc.edu/vrml
Community Place	http://sonypic.com/vs
WIRL	http://www.vream.com

Chat

ichat	http://www.ichat.com

News services

Pointcast	http://www.pointcast.com
Castanet	http://www.marimba.com
News Ticker	http://www.netcontrols.com

Search Utilities

AnySearch	http://www.privnet.com

Web Authoring Programs

Hot Dog	http://www.sausage.com

Programming

ActiveX	http://www.microsoft.com
Java	http://www.sun.com

D Bibliography and Online Resources

Everything has been said before, but since nobody listens we have to keep going back and beginning all over again.

André Gide

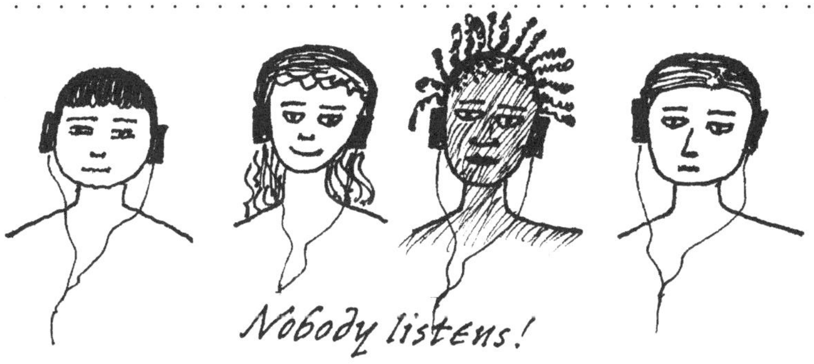

You won't learn to use a computer by reading a book; hands-on practice is necessary. Books give additional details, however. In general computer books more than two years old or Internet books more than one year old are the equivalent of grammar books from the last century: outdated. Essays and dictionaries last a little longer.

Bookstores and Distributors

(Links available at http://NewWindPub.com/workbook)

You can order medical books directly from most medical distributors.

J.A. Majors	http://www.majors.com	(800) 241-6551
Login Brothers (institutions only)	http://www.lb.com	(800) 621-4249
Matthews Medical Books	http://www.mattmccoy.com	(800) 633-2665
Springhouse	http://www.springnet.com	(800) 666-5597

If you need to find a publisher's Web site, go to: http://www.lights.com/publisher

You can also order general interest books directly on the Web from Amazon, Barnes and Noble, and Bookserve. BookWeb maintains a searchable list of bookstores both in the USA and abroad.

Amazon	http://www.amazon.com
Barnes and Noble	http://www.barnesandnoble.com
Bookserve	http://www.bookserve.com
BookWeb	http://www.bookweb.org/directory

Recommended Books (in order)

- *Teach Yourself Computers and the Internet Visually* (Maran, 1996)
- *Web Search Strategies* (Pfaffenberger, 1996)
- *The Internet Book* (Comer, 1995)
- *The Trouble With Computers* (Landauer, 1995)
- *Data Smog* (Shenk, 1997)

Computer Journals and Books

Online computer journals, most with full text. These are an excellent resource for all things computing and Internet. Journals that cover advanced topics (such as programming) are not listed here.

Byte	http://www.byte.com
Computer Currents	http://www.currents.net
Computers in Nursing	http://www.cini.com/cin/cin.htm
HomePC	http://www.homepc.com
Internet World	http://www.iw.com
On the Internet	http://www.isoc.org
PC Computing	http://www.zdnet.com/pccomp
PC Magazine Online	http://www.pcmag.com
Que Bookshelf (40 complete books)	http://www.mcp.com/que/bookshelf
PC World	http://www.pcworld.com
Windows 95 Magazine	http://www.win95mag.com
Windows Magazine	http://www.winmag.com
ZDNet	http://www.zdnet.com

BIBLIOGRAPHY

Ackermann, Ernest. (1995). *Learning to Use the Internet.* Wilsonville : Frank Beedle & Associates.
Dated, but if you are using command-line programs (Pine, Pico, Lynx) this book has step-by-step instructions.

Altman, Russ. (1997). Informatics in the care of patients: ten notable challenges. *Western Journal of Medicine* (166) 2:118-122.
Short, non-technical discussion of the future of medicine and computers.

Anthony, Denis. (1996). *Health on the Internet.* London : Blackwell Science
Good introduction. Academic, teaching, international focus.

Arntson et al. (1997). *Learning the Internet.* New York : DDC Publishing.
A workbook, with exercises, covering basic Internet topics.

Barry, John A. (1991). *Technobabble.* Cambridge : MIT Press.
A wonderful analysis of the current state of computer language: obscure, over-heated, and vague.

Berinstein, Paula. (1996). *Finding Images Online.* Wilton, CT : Pemberton Press.
Also explains how to download them, what the different types are, etc.

Bernzweig, Eli P. (1990). The Nurse's Liability for Malpractice : A Programmed Course. St. Louis, Mo. : C.V. Mosby Co.

Brande, Dorothea. (1934). *Becoming a Writer.* Los Angeles : Jeremy Tarcher.
One of a kind. There is more practical wisdom in this book than any ten other books on writing.

Cassagne, Hervé. (1997). *Internet pour les Médecins, 2ème* ed. : Editions Médicales Spécialisées.
Workbook similar to this one, by an Internet trainer and journalist in Paris.

Comer, Douglas E. (1995). *The Internet Book.* Englewood Cliffs: Prentice Hall.
Probably the best explanation you can find about the Internet. Clearly written, well illustrated.

Edwards, Margaret J. A. (1997). *The Internet for Nurses and Allied Health Professionals.* New York : Springer Verlag.
Almost the same as *The Internet for Physicians* that she co-wrote with Smith. Emphasis on Usenet, mailing lists.

Forester, Tom and Morrison, Perry. (1994). *Computer Ethics.* Cambridge : MIT Press.

Duboff, Leonard. (1992). *The Law (in Plain English) for Writers.* New York : Wiley.

Duboff, Leonard. (1993). *The Law (in Plain English) for Health Care Professionals.* New York : Wiley.

Forsyth, David. (1997). Searching for Digital Pictures. *Scientific American.* June (276) 6.

Goldstein, Douglas and Flory, Joyce. *The Online Guide to Healthcare & Wellness.* Irwin Professional Publishing.

Goldstein, Douglas and Flory, Joyce. (1997) *The Online Guide to Healthcare Management & Medicine.* Irwin Professional Publishing.

Hancock, Lee. (1996). *Physicians' Guide to the Internet.* Philadelphia: Lippincott-Raven
Short introduction, followed by an annotated list of sites, many of them mailing lists.

Hannah, Kathryn and Hall, Marion, Eds. (1995). *Nursing Informatics* (2nd ed.). New York : Springer-Verlag.
Textbookish. Approach with caution.

Heslop, Brent and Angell, David. (1994). *The Instant Internet Guide.* Reading : Addison-Wesley.

Hoben, John. (1997). *1997 Guide to Health Care Resources on the Internet.* Faulkner and Gray.

Hoffman, Paul. (1996). *The Internet Instant Reference.* 3rd Ed. San Francisco : Sybex.
A glossary-style reference. Short and to the point.

Hogarth, Michael and Hutchinson, David. (1996). *An Internet Guide for the Health Professional.* (2nd ed.). Sacramento : New Wind Publishing.

Hutchinson, David. (1997). *A Pocket Guide to the Medical Internet.* (2nd ed.). Sacramento : New Wind Publishing.
A reference to medical sites, directories, and indices. Also search engines, directories. By specialty.

Kiley, Robert. (1996). *Medical Information on the Internet.* Edinburgh : Churchill Livingstone.

Jenders, Sideli, Hripcsak. (1996). *Introduction to Medical Informatics.* Columbia University. [Online]: http://www.cpmc.columbia/edu/textbook

Landauer, Thomas K. (1995). *The Trouble with Computers : Usefulness, Usability, and Productivity.* Cambridge : MIT Press.
Excellent analysis, in non-technical language, of the sad state of computers. Practical adjunct to Stoll's sobering thoughts on the Internet.

Li, X. & Crane, N.B. (1996). *Electronic Styles: A Handbook for Citing Electronic Information.* Medford : Information Today.

Linden, Dr. Tom. (1995). *Dr. Tom Linden's Guide to Online Medicine.* New York : McGraw-Hill.
Short book. The medical Internet has come a long way since 1995.

Maran. (1996). *Teach Yourself Computers and the Internet Visually.* Foster City : Maran Graphics.
Excellent introduction. Highly recommended. Full-color graphics, simple definitions.

McKenzie, Bruce C. (1996). *Medicine and the Internet: Introducing Online Resources and Terminology.* Oxford, New York: Oxford University.
Decent, but already dated, and written in academic jargon.

Moran, Richard. (1994). *Beware Those Who Ask for Feedback.* New York : HarperBusiness

Moran, Richard. (1993). *Never Confuse A Memo With Reality.* New York : HarperBusiness

Negroponte, Nicholas. (1995). *Being Digital.* New York : Knopf.

Nicoll, Leslie H. (1997). *Nurses' Guide to the Internet.* Philadelphia : Lippincott-Raven.
Short introduction, list of sites. Emphasis on mailing lists.

Osheroff, Jerome A. (1995). *Computers in Clinical Practice.* Philadelphia : American College of Physicians.
All-around introduction to computers and medicine, including medical records, decision support, and office management.

Pareras, Luis G. M.D. (1996). *Medicine and the Internet.* Boston : Little, Brown and Company.
Oversize book (640 pages). Buy a standard Internet text instead.

Pence, Gregory. (1995). *Classic Cases In Medical Ethics.* 2nd Ed. New York : McGraw-Hill

Saba, Virginia and McCormick, Kathleen. (1996). *Essentials of Computers for Nurses.* (2nd ed.). New York : McGraw-Hill.
A relatively friendly introduction to computers; physicians will find this useful also.

Mendelson, Edward. (1997). Off-line search utilities. *PC Magazine,* (16) 7, 227-232.

Mendelson, Edward. (1997) Off-line browsers, PC Magazine (16) 7, 207-218.

Mullet, Kevin and Sano, Darrell. (1995). *Designing Visual Interfaces : Communication Oriented Techniques.* Englewood Cliffs, NJ : SunSoft Press.
Highly recommended if you are creating a Web page, or anything else.

Munro, Kathryn. (1997). Internet filtering utilities. *PC Magazine* (16) 7, 235-240

Pfaffenberger, Bryan. (1997). *Protect Your Privacy on the Internet.* New York : John Wiley and Sons
Practical, easy to understand. Covers simple matters (filling out forms) as well as technical ones (PGP).

Pfaffenberger, Bryan. (1996) Web Search Strategies. New York : MIS Press.

Postman, Neil. (1985). *Amusing Ourselves to Death: Public Discourse in the Age of Show Business.* New York: Viking Penguin.

Ryer, Jeanne C. (1997). *Health Net.* New York : John Wiley and Sons.
Brief introduction to health resources on the Internet, written for the consumer. Limited number of sites listed.

Shenk, David. (1997) *Data Smog: Surviving the Information Age.* New York : Harper Collins.
Critical book about the current computer and Internet frenzy. If you're feeling frazzled, read this book.

Smith, Roger P., MD, and Edwards, Margaret J.A. (1997). *The Internet for Physicians.* New York : Springer Verlag.
Short book. Introduction to the internet. Half the book (60 pages) is the list of sites.

Stoll, Clifford. (1995). *Silicon Snake Oil: Second Thoughts on the Information Highway.* New York : Doubleday.
Healthy doubts about the point of it all. From the author of *The Cuckoo's Egg.*

Turkle, Sherry. (1995). *Life on the Screen: Identity in the Age of the Internet.* New York : Simon and Schuster.

Weinman, Lynda. (1996). *Designing Web Graphics.* Indianapolis : New Riders.

Weizenbaum, Joseph. (1976). *Computer Power and Human Reason.* San Francisco : W.H.Freeman.
Convincing arguments about what makes us human, and them mechanical.

Wilson, Ralph. (1991). *Help! The Art of Computer Technical Support.* Berkeley : Peachpit Press.
Practical instructions on planning for, delivering, and evaluating support.

E Glossary

'Twas brillig, and the slithy toves
Did gyre and gimble in the wabe;
All mimsy were the borogoves,
And the mome raths outgrabe.

Lewis Carroll, Alice In Wonderland

Until computers become truly friendly, you will often need to consult a dictionary to work with them. No doubt at least once you will have to explain a computer problem or question over the telephone, where knowing the right word can mean the difference between success and failure.

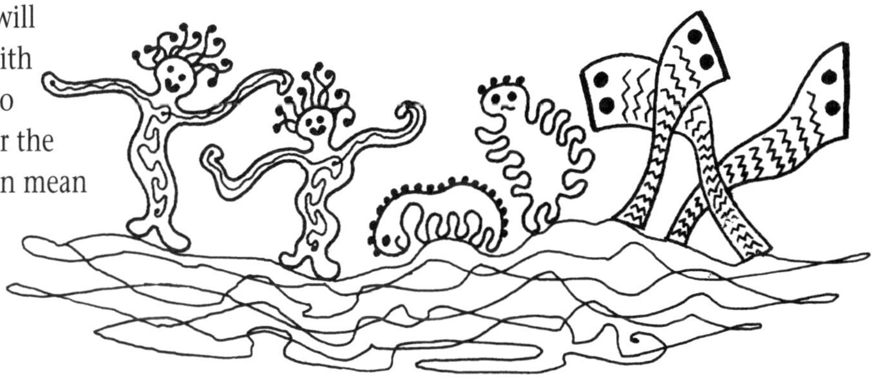

The Essential List of Computer and Internet Words to Understand

browser	hypertext	program
cursor	icon	scroll bar
database	Internet	search engine
directory	mailing list	URL
disk	menu	window
email	online	word processor
file	operating system	World Wide Web
home page	password	

Terms not included:

- health agencies (NIH, CDC, NIDDK)
- Internet agencies (IETF, IAB)
- electrical and engineering terms (twisted pair, FDDI)
- Greek, Sanskrit, tekspeak, and bitbabble

Online Computer Glossaries

(Links available at http://NewWindPub.com/workbook)

Computers and Health Care	http://www.acl.lanl.gov/sunrise/Medical/ota/16appg.txt
Computers, Networking	http://www-med.stanford.edu/center/mednet/glossary.html
Computers	http://www.sandybay.com/pc-web
Computers; technical	http://www.rirr.cnuce.cnr.it/Glossario/glhpage.html
Computers	http://wfn-shop.Princeton.edu/foldoc
DOS terms	http://www.csulb.edu/~murdock/easydos.html
Computer Encyclopedia	http://whatis.com
Hacker's Dictionary	http://www.ccil.org/jargon/jargon_toc.html
Health Care Cybervision	http://www.hccybervision.com/glossary.html
Internet Reference	http://www.msn.com/tutorial/glossary.html
Internet terms	http://www.matisse.net/files/glossary.html
Technical Encyclopedia	http://www.techweb.com/encyclopedia/defineterm.cgi

286, 386, 486
Naming scheme for PC computers before the Pentium. The numbers refer to the type of processor in the computer.

32 bit, 16 bit
Number of pieces of information that an operating system or a program can work with. Windows 95 is a 32-bit operating system, whereas Windows 3.1 is 16-bit.

A

abstract
Summary of an article. MEDLINE and CINAHL include abstracts.

accessory
Small program designed for a limited function, such as a calculator or clock.

ADT
Admission, Discharge, Transfer. System that tracks patients as they are admitted, leave, or move from area to area in a hospital.

advocacy
Working on behalf of another; trying to help a person by acting as a go-between with an organization, or to obtain a service.

alias
Short, easy to remember name that is used instead of a longer or more difficult one. Many email programs let you type an alias into the address line; they then substitute the full address when sending the message.

algorithm
Formula for solving a problem. Algorithms are widely used in many fields, including clinical medicine and nursing.

analog
Information expressing a continuous amount of a physical quantity. A mercury thermometer and sweep watch display analog information of temperature and time. See *digital.*

annotation
Short note or review. Directories may have annotations beside each link, describing what you will find on that Web page.

applet
Small Java program that is sent along with a Web page.

application
A (relatively large) computer program.

archie
Function on the Internet for finding FTP files.

archive
Collection of past information or records.

article
Posting on a newsgroup.

attachment
File that is sent along with an email message.

avatar
1. Incarnation of God in the Hindu religion.
2. Icon that you choose for yourself when navigating a virtual reality scene.

B

backbone
Internet trunk lines between major points.

backup
To make a second copy of files on a physically different medium (disk or tape), so that if something happens to the original computer you will still have the information.

bandwidth
Amount of information a cable or medium can carry measured in bits per second. See *T-1.*

banner
Advertisement on a Web site, usually rectangular, often with animated text or graphics.

bcc
Blind Carbon Copy. An email function whereby the addresses of the persons you send it to are hidden. See *cc, reply to all.*

binary
1. Mathematical scheme which computers use to represent information at their most fundamental level. A binary symbol is either 1 or 0.
2. Program files (as opposed to text files). These are transferred in binary format when sent from one computer to another.

bit
A binary digit, 0 or 1. Digital computers store information as bits. Eight bits equals one byte. Programs, files, and drive space are measured in bytes. See *kilobyte, megabyte, gigabyte, terabyte.*

boot, re-boot
To start or re-start a computer.

Boolean logic
Use of the words and, or, and and not to narrow or broaden a search.

brain dump
Telling everything you know about a subject.

broadcasting
Sending information out, such as on the radio or television, where any device which uses that medium can receive it. See *multicasting.*

browser
Program for reading documents on the World Wide Web, such as Netscape.

browsing
1. Searching by MeSH word in order to look at related categories for a concept.
2. Moving around on the Internet without a specific goal in mind, similar to browsing the shelves of a bookstore or library.

bulletin board system (BBS)
Locally-run computer system that people can dial into to exchange files, make announcements, or carry on discussions.

Butterfly effect
Phenomenon of complex systems whereby a small initial condition causes a large and unpredictable effect after a period of time.

button
1. Small, usually rectangular onscreen area that you click with the mouse pointer to activate a function.
2. Physical button, such as on a mouse.

button bar
Group of onscreen icons found along the top or bottom of a program window or Web page.

byte
Group of (usually eight) bits that represents one letter or number in a computer.

C

card
See *network card.*

case sensitivity
Treating capital and lower-case letters as different. For example, in a case-sensitive search, java and Java will give different results.

catalog
Library science: a listing of books or articles.

cc
Carbon Copy. Sending a copy of a message to another person at the same time as the original is sent. See *bcc, reply to all.*

CD-ROM (CD)
Compact Disc/Read-Only Media. Current CD's hold 650,000 bytes, but larger capacity ones will be available in a few years. Compact discs are now being made which can be recorded several times.

cell
One box in a spreadsheet where a number, text, or formula can be placed.

censorship
Official suppression of information.

cgi
Common Gateway Interface. A standard that allows a browser to invoke a program which is running on a Web server. For example, the program can connect with a database and return the results to the browser.

chart
Graphical representation of numerical information as a pie, bar, or line.

chat
Conference connection on the Internet where several people type or talk together. Before Web-based chat, this was done through Internet Relay Chat.

check box
Square area on a screen which you click to make a choice; you can check more than one. See *radio button.*

CINAHL
Cumulative Index to Nursing and Allied Health Literature.

citation
1. Listing or record in a library catalog.
2. Listing in the bibliography.
3. Quotation or mention of something.

client
Computer or program that makes a request of a server, usually over the Internet. A World Wide Web browser is a client program which requests Web pages.

clinical information system
A computer system (hardware and software) that handles most or all clinical information in a hospital and clinics.

clip art
Images that you can use in a publication. Before computer clip art became available, you had to purchase a book of clip art, then cut out an image for your publication.

closed list
Mailing list which you must request to join; subscription is not automated.

command-line
Way of interacting with a computer (interface) which requires you to enter keyboard commands to activate programs or features. See *graphical user interface.*

compression
Using a computer program to reduce the size of a file so that it can be sent more quickly or take up less space in storage.

confidentiality
Principle that communication between a patient and a healthcare professional is private and not to be shared with the public. This applies to written information, such as the medical record.

configuration
Way in which a particular piece of hardware or software is set up.

consumer health
Information for patients or the public.

controlled vocabulary
Using a standard vocabulary for a subject, rather than allowing non-standard or colloquial terms.

cookie
Piece of information sent by a Web server to a browser, which can be used for login or registration, or to keep other information. See *browser, server.*

copyright
Author's or artist's right to control the use of what is created, in order to prevent others from copying the work. Often referred to as intellectual property rights.

CPU
Central Processing Unit; the chip that does the main work in a computer. Also called processor, microprocessor, chip.

cracker
Person who tries to illegally enter, or "crack into" a computer. See *hacker.*

cursor
Blinking line or box on a computer screen; if you type, that is where the letters will appear.

cyberspace
Term for the Internet coined by William Gibson in his 1984 novel, *Neuromancer.*

D

database
Program or the resulting file that structures information by categories. A typical hospital has a patient database.

daybook
Small book for noting a day's appointments.

decision support
Computer program to help make decisions. For example, it may present possible diagnoses based on a patient's symptoms.

dedicated connection
Connection to the Internet that is always available to the computer; these computers are usually on a network. See *dialup connection.*

defamatory
Statement that subjects a person or institution to hatred, contempt or ridicule, or one that results in injury to his business or work reputation.

default
Initial settings for a program, equivalent to factory settings for equipment.

defragment
Process of rearranging the files on a hard drive. Files become fragmented over time, slowing down your computer. DOS and Windows have defragmenting programs.

desktop
Visual arrangement of the main computer screen, which includes such things as the Windows 95 start button, program icons, or a taskbar.

desktop publishing
Program that can layout text and graphics for publication.

dialup connection
Connection to the Internet made through a modem by dialing a service provider. See *dedicated connection.*

dialog box
Window that gives you choices for a specific function such as printing.

DICOM
Digital and Communications in Medicine. A standard for encoding and retrieving medical images, such as x-rays or CT scans.

digest
Summary of information. On a mailing list you can receive digests of messages sent, rather than receive each message as it comes in. The digest may be sent weekly, or when it reaches a certain size.

digital
Composed of discrete quantities. Modern computers save all information as binary digits, ones and zeros. See *analog.*

directory
1. Sub-section of a computer's files for holding or organizing other files.
2. Subject-based listing of sites available on the Internet.

disclosure
In medicine, the idea that a patient is informed of all the relevant information related to the disease or treatment. See *informed consent.*

discussion group
Electronic forum on the Usenet where people post comments and questions.

disk
Physical mechanism for storing information. A floppy disk holds 1.4 to 2.8 megabytes. See *memory, CD-ROM, hard disk.*

distributed computing
Information or functions distributed among computers that are physically separate.

document delivery service
Company that supplies copies of articles.

domain name
Name (e.g. nih.gov) used to find a computer on the Internet. Domain names are purchased from InterNIC.

double-click
To click the left mouse button twice in quick succession.

download
To transfer text or pictures from a distant computer to the computer in front of you.

drag and drop
To click an item, such as a bookmark, drag it across the screen to another location, then drop it there by releasing the mouse button.

drunk mouse syndrome
When the mouse pointer starts jumping erratically around the screen.

dweeb
Geek wanna-be.

E

EMR
Electronic Medical Record. Integrated system that collects and manages medical information, including monitor data, flow charts, and narrative information.

email
Electronic mail.

encryption
Process of coding information to make it secure so it cannot be intercepted or read by an unauthorized person.

error
Temporary problem in a computer. Euphemistically called bugs, glitches, faults.

ethics
Study of what a person or group ought to do; what actions are morally right.

exact match
Option in searching. To specify that a search engine look for an exact word or phrase.

expert system
Computer program that uses reasoning or rules to help solve problems.

Explorer (Internet)
Internet Explorer is Microsoft's browser, whereas Explorer is their program for managing files.

export
To take information from one document or program and save it in another format.

F

fact sheet
Short description of something. In medicine, often a handout written for the public.

fair use
Use of small portions of a copyrighted work "for purposes such as criticism, comment, news reporting, teaching (including multiple copies for classroom use), scholarship or research" (Copyright Act of 1976).

fax
Short for facsimile. A way of graphically copying a page and sending it over a telephone line.

FAQ
Frequently Asked Questions. Really, answers to these questions, often in the form of an introduction to a topic or group.

fields
Categories a database uses to organize information. In searching, you can often choose to search for a word in a particular field such as title, name, subject, or journal.

file
Any document (text, picture, database, spreadsheet) saved in a computer.

filter
Automatic function used in email to sort incoming mail according to who it came from, the subject of the message, etc. In general, sorting information.

firewall
Computer placed between an institution's networks and the Internet to prevent security breaches of the institution's computer systems.

flame
An angry statement sent by email.

floppy (disk)
Small rectangular disk used to store files, or transfer them from one computer to another.

follow-up
1) Replying to a post on a newsgroup.
2) Continuing the action started, such as calling a person after a meeting.
3) Re-examination of a patient after the first meeting.

font
Size and style of written text. For example, the entries in this glossary are size 10, bold, in Stone Serif.

form
Text boxes and buttons on a screen for entering information. With spreadsheet and database programs you can create forms.

format
1. Look of text on paper or screen.
2. Coding for a type of information. Most programs save files in a particular format.
3. To reset the basic logical structure of a disk, thereby erasing all its information.

formula
Algebraic sequence of numbers and variables in the cell of a spreadsheet for performing automatic calculations. See *function*.

forum
Place for public discussion. On the Internet, commonly done with the Usenet.

frame
Rectangular area on a Web site containing a separate Web page, often for a navigation bar.

freeware
Free software.

fritterware
Program that fritters away your time.

FTP
File Transfer Protocol. Protocol on the Internet that enables rapid transfer of files from one computer to another.

full-text search
Searching the complete text of a document, compared with searching limited sections such as the title.

function
Ready-to-use formula in a spreadsheet.

G

geek
Person who actually enjoys working with computers. Formerly pejorative. Variants: nerd, wuss, chip-head, turbo-nerd.

gigabyte
One billion bytes, abbreviated as GB. See *bit.*

gigaflop
One billion floating point operations per second.

gopher
Protocol on the Internet that enables menu-style choices. Gopher immediately preceded the World Wide Web, and was very popular for a few years.

graphic
Picture on a computer, as opposed to text.

GUI
Graphical User Interface. A computer system that has pictures, menus, and onscreen buttons. See *command-line interface.*

grok
To understand globally or intimately.

H

hacker
Person whose approach to programming is the quick-fix, rather than a disciplined approach. See *cracker.*

handshaking
Two devices connecting to one another. The screeching you hear when a modem connects to another modem is one kind of handshaking.

hard disk
Main disk inside a computer that stores information in magnetic form.

header
Information at the top of a document or message. Web pages and email messages have headers with different kinds of information.

helper application
Program that runs alongside your browser to extend its capabilities, for example to play sounds, animations, or video. See *plug-in.*

hierarchies
System of classification. The levels of a Usenet group are shown by dots: sci.med.nursing

HIS
Hospital Information System. Traditional name for a mainframe-based system with patient and financial data. Historically, a HIS handles only limited types of information, unlike a true Electronic Medical Record.

HL-7
Health Level 7. A standard for coding patient information which enables different departments, hospitals and institutions to exchange information electronically.

home page
The opening or main Web page for a person, institution, or business.

host
Computer on a network that supplies communication services such as email, gopher, FTP, telnet, or the Web.

host name
Name of a computer on the Internet, such as www.nih.gov

hotline
Telephone number you call for information.

hypertext
Document with computer-activated links to other documents. On the Web a hypertext link shows up as an underlined word; you click it to make the jump to the next document.

HTML
HyperText Markup Language. The coding used to create documents for the Web.

HTTP
HyperText Transport Protocol. The protocol that transmits hypertext-style documents.

I

ICD-9
International Classification of Diseases, #9 Disease hierarchy from the World Health Organization. Now used for billing.

icon
Small picture signifying a program, file, or function.

identifier
Every citation in MEDLINE has a number assigned to it, called its Unique Identifier, or UID, which you can search for.

imagemap
Picture in a document with areas you can click to jump to other documents.

import
To bring information into a document from another file or document. With Netscape you can import another person's bookmark list.

index
Catalog or database of citations, which may include listings by author, title, and subject.

indexing
Method used by a search engine to compile a database of words found in Internet sites.

informatics (medical or nursing)
Study of computers related to health care.

informed consent
Idea that a patient fully understands a treatment before consenting to it. See *disclosure*.

interface
Way a computer program interacts with you, for example through onscreen buttons or keyboard commands. The two most common interfaces are graphical user interface and command-line interface.

intranet
Network designed to exchange information within an organization using TCP/IP.

Internet
Worldwide collection of networks that communicate with each other using TCP/IP.

Internet II
Project funded by the government and 100 universities to set up a research and educational network for testing new protocols and high-speed bandwidth. Started 1996.

Internet account
Service you get from an Internet service provider. May include access to the Internet, an email box, and a Web page.

Internet service provider
Company that sells access to the Internet, usually for a monthly fee.

Internet Worm, the Great
Worm set loose in 1988 that brought hundreds of Internet computers to their knees.

IP address
Addressing scheme used by the Internet. Each computer or device has a unique 32-bit IP address, four 8-bit numbers each of which can be 0-256. The total number of addresses can thus be a little more than 4 billion. A new standard is being developed (IPv6) which will have 128 bits. The total number of addresses will then be 3.4×10^{38}, or about 6 billion billion addresses per square yard of the earth.

ISDN
Integrated Services Digital Network. A type of connection which can send/receive information at 128 kilobits/second.

J

Java
Programming language on the Web that allows small programs (applets) to be sent with a Web page and run on your computer.

Jazz drive
Drive with disks similar to a floppy. Each disk can hold one gigabyte of data. Useful for archiving data or backing up a hard drive.

K

keyword search
Searching for words which have been entered into the keyword field for a document. This is often a better way to find documents related to a subject than a full-text search.

kilobyte
A thousand bytes, abbreviated as KB. See *bit*.

L

laptop
Portable computer that can fit on your lap. Notebook and palmtop computers are smaller.

layout
1. General arrangement of pictures and words on a page or screen.
2. Specific properties of a printed page such as margins, paper size, headers, or line numbering.

liability
Being responsible for harm done to another person. A professional can be held liable for negligence by failing to uphold a standard of conduct for his profession. See *negligence, professional relationship*.

libel
Published statement defamatory towards another person or institution. See *slander*.

link
Word or picture in a hypertext document that you click to jump to another document.

listproc
One program which runs a mailing list.

listserv
Most common type of program that runs a mailing list.

LAN
Local Area Network. A network serving a limited area such as one building. A LAN has a central file server connected to a number of desktop computers called workstations.

login
Name you use when you access a computer along with a password. See *security*.

logout
Entering a command such as "exit" to break your connection with a network.

lurking
Silent participation in a mailing list or other group: reading messages but not contributing.

lynx
Text-only browser used on UNIX computers.

M

mailbox
Place where email is stored. You have a personal box on your service provider's computer. When you check your email, it is downloaded to the inbox on your PC.

mailing list
Automated way for a group of people to communicate with each other via email. See *listserv, listproc.*

mainframe
Central computer with large storage and a fast CPU, connected to a variety of peripheral terminals. A mainframe computer typically contains a large database.

mandelbug
Problem whose underlying cause is so complex that it appears random or chaotic.

marking
With a newsreader program, you can "mark" a newsgroup, thread, or message as already read, so you won't see it in a list anymore.

MEDLARS
Set of databases from the National Library of Medicine with information related to medical practice and research. Includes MEDLINE, TOXNET, AIDSLINE, and others.

MEDLINE
Online database of medical citations from the National Library of Medicine.

megabyte
One million bytes, abbreviated as MB. See *bit.*

megahertz
Millions of cycles per second. A measure of computer speed; for example, a P166 is a Pentium with a speed of 166 megahertz.

memory
RAM, Random Access Memory. Where programs are stored while they run.

menu
List of choices that appears when you click an onscreen word. Most programs have a menu bar with File, Edit, and Help menu items.

MeSH
Medical Subject Headings. The terminology used by the National Library of Medicine for Index Medicus and MEDLINE.

meta-
One level higher in abstraction.

metadirectory
List of directories.

metasearch
Program that takes your word and looks at several search engines rather than just one.

metathesaurus
Format that integrates more than 30 biomedical vocabularies, containing information about concepts, the classifications used, relationships among terms, etc.

microcomputer, minicomputer
Older terms for small or mid-level computers. As desktop CPU's become more powerful, these terms are less meaningful.

MIME
Multipurpose Internet Mail Extensions. The standard for attaching non-text files (such as a graphic picture) to an email message.

modem
A modulator/demodulator card or device which converts digital information into a form that can travel over the telephone line, where another modem converts the information.

moderator
Person who reads mailing list messages first to decide whether they will be posted. Subscriptions can also be moderated. See *closed list.*

monitor
The TV-like box with the computer screen.

mouse
Small device which you push across a pad to control the onscreen pointer.

multicasting
Sending information directly to multiple computers or recipients. A postal letter which goes to one person could be called unicasting, while radio or TV is broadcasting.

multimedia
Any kind of information other than text, such as pictures, animation, sound, and video.

N

natural language processing
Ability of a computer to understand common (natural) language, rather than special commands or computer languages.

navigation bar
Row of icons on a Web site that points to the main areas of that site. Navigation bars are often within a frame.

negligence
Failing to act in a reasonable and prudent manner. See *liability.*

nesting
Placing containers within containers, such as a bookmark folder within another bookmark folder.

Netscape Navigator
Most popular browser program for the World Wide Web.

network
Two or more computers which are connected together in order to send information back and forth. Most existing networks use a proprietary protocol such as Netware, but companies are now setting up intranets that use the TCP/IP protocol. See also: *local area network.*

network card
Physical card in a computer that the computer uses to send information over a network.

news server
Internet computer which carries messages for Usenet newsgroups.

newsgroup
Computerized bulletin-board.

newsreader
Program for reading Usenet newsgroups. Netscape includes a newsreader program.

nicknames
Term Eudora uses for email aliases.

nursing practice act
Law enacted in each state that defines the limits of professional nursing practice.

O

ODBC
Open DataBase Connect. A language used to move data into or out of a database based on SQL.

offline
Anything done while not connected to a network. Most email programs let you download messages quickly, then disconnect in order to read offline.

online
Anything you do while connected to a network, such as browsing or searching a database.

operating system
Underlying program that runs the basic functions on a computer. Macintosh, UNIX, and Windows are different operating systems.

P

packet switching
Method used to send information on the Internet. Data is broken up into packets, each of which has the destination address. A packet is directed by computers called routers, and each packet travels independently.

PACS
Picture Archiving and Communication System. A computerized system for collecting, archiving and displaying images.

password
Secret word that you use to gain access to a computer or network. Passwords are the main mechanism for computer security. See *login*.

PC
Personal Computer. A computer that an average person can afford.

phrase search
Searching for a complete phrase rather than individual words.

pixel
Picture Element. The smallest area on a computer screen.

port
1. Connection on the back of a computer for a device such as a modem, mouse, keyboard, or monitor.
2. Settings within the computer.

PCMCIA
Personal Computer Memory Card International Association. Standard for credit-card sized slots and devices for laptop computers, such as a removable modem, hard drive, or video device.

PDF
Portable Document Format. Common format for non-HTML documents on the Web.

peer review
Having other professionals (peers) review written materials in order to certify that the information is authoritative or correct.

plug-in
Program integrated with a Web browser to extend its capabilities, for example to play sounds, animations, or video. See *helper application*.

point-of-care
System (such as a hand-held computer) that enables staff to enter information into an electronic medical record at the time they are giving care.

POP
Post Office Protocol. A protocol used for electronic mail. POP is used to read mail, whereas SMTP is used to send it.

posting
Sending an email message to a public area, such as a mailing list or newsgroup.

program
Series of instructions for a computer to carry out. Synonyms: software, applications, utilities, code, accessories, binaries, or executables.

properties
Aspects of a file, message, document, or other computer object.

PPP
Point to Point Protocol. Used for connecting to the Internet via a modem.

privacy
Keeping something out of public view; secret.

professional relationship
Relationship between a healthcare professional and a patient, created when the professional provides care for that person. See *liability*, *negligence*.

professional responsibility
Requirement that a licensed professional act as another reasonable and prudent person would who has the same training, experience, and skills.

protocol
Description of the rules that two computers use to exchange information.

proximity search
Function on some search engines that allows you to look for a word if it appears near another word, for example in the same sentence or paragraph.

proxy server
Computer that acts as an intermediary server. A company can set up a proxy server between desktop computers and the Internet which will filter traffic, store information, and monitor attempts to breach security.

push technology
Information being sent to you. Web browsing is pull; multicasting or broadcasting is push.

Q

query
Automated question on a database. For example, "How many patients ages 25-45, who were admitted in June with a diagnosis of head trauma, stayed longer than three days?"

R

radio button
Circular image on the screen that you click to choose that option. If there are several radio buttons in a group, you can choose only one. See *check box.*

RAM
Random Access Memory. Electronic chips used to store programs while they are in use.

ranking
Displaying the results of a search with the sites listed (ranked) in order of the best match to your search word or phrase.

real time
Occurring at the same time, concurrent, as opposed to delayed. Chat rooms function in real time; email does not.

re-boot
Restart a computer.

record
Information on one item in a database. For example, all the information on one patient (name, address, unit number) constitutes one record. In MEDLINE, all the information on one article or book is one record.

reference
See *citation.*

registry
File in Windows 95 where all information is stored about the system and programs.

reply to all
Function of email programs whereby you respond to everyone who received the message. See *bcc, cc.*

return address
Email address which is sent along with a message as part of the header.

return receipt
Optional function of email programs. If you send a message with this turned on, you will get an automatic message back when the other person opens your note.

right-clicking
Clicking the right mouse button. In Windows 95 this causes a menu to pop up with choices related to the item you clicked.

router
Computer on the Internet which forwards packets. It examines the address of each incoming packet and determines the best route to reach its destination.

S

scanning
Using a machine (a scanner) to read text or images from a printed page and convert to digital information. OCR (Optical Character Recognition) is software that recognizes text.

scroll bar
Rectangular bar that appears in a window when there is more information than will fit in the space. When you click in the scroll bar, the information scrolls down the screen.

search engine
Internet site where you search for information that is available on the Internet.

security
Hardware and software to protect data and hardware from (intentional or unintentional) harm. This can include passwords, proxy servers, firewalls, encryption, and other methods. See *SSL, proxy.*

server
Computer or software that serves information to a requesting computer (client) using a particular protocol such as HTTP, gopher, FTP.

service provider
Company that sells access to the Internet.

set
Collection of items. In MEDLINE you can save the results of a search as a set, in order to look at those results later.

shareware
Computer program that is available for a free trial period.

shell account
Account that gives you access to a computer running Internet software with the UNIX operating system, a command-line interface.

shortcut
Visual item in Windows 95 that points to a file, program, or drive. Shortcuts can be arranged on the desktop or in folders.

signature
Automatic lines that an email program can put at the bottom of each message, with your name, email address, etc.

slander
Defamatory statement that is spoken aloud rather than written. See *libel.*

SLIP
Serial Line Internet Protocol. A phone connection for using the Web with a graphical browser such as Netscape. See *PPP.*

smart card
Credit-card sized device with built-in computer memory or programs.

smiley
Face-drawing created by keyboard symbols, used to indicate emotions.

SMS
Shared Medical Systems. A company that sells mainframe medical information systems.

SMTP
Simple Mail Transport Protocol. The protocol for sending email.

SNOMED
Systematized Nomenclature of Medicine. Classification scheme put together by the College of American Pathologists with seven axes: topology, morphology, etiology, function, disease, procedure, and occupation.

software
Computer program.

spamming
Sending unwanted email to a large number of people. Done with mailing lists, newsgroups, or special bulk email programs.

speech recognition
Ability of a computer to understand or transcribe spoken words.

spelling checker
Function that examines a document for spelling errors and suggests correct spelling. Can be set to make corrections as you type.

spreadsheet
Program for making automatic calculations and graphs.

SQL
Structured Query Language. International standard language for defining and making inquiries of a relational database. See *ODBC.*

SSL
Secure Sockets Layer. Protocol that allows sensitive information to be sent safely. Uses a Security Certificate with a unique number to identify each person. See *security.*

startup disk
Floppy disk used to start your computer if a problem occurs with the hard drive.

streaming
Sound or video that starts to play as soon as it arrives to your browser, rather than waiting until the entire file is downloaded.

subject line
Line that gives the topic of an email message.

subscribing
Signing up for a journal or other periodical information.

suite
Group of programs sold together, such as a word processor, spreadsheet, and database.

surfing
Slang term for moving from document to document on the World Wide Web.

surveillance
Watching over a person or spying on him.

T

T-1
Type of line that carries 1.54 megabits of information/second. Ethernet (T-10) carries 10 megabits/second; T-3 carries 44.7. See *bandwidth.*

TCP/IP
Transmission Control Protocol/Internet Protocol. Underlying software which sends each Internet message as a series of packets.

technobabble
What you see and hear in computer books, conventions, and stores.

techspeak
Coherent technobabble.

tele-
At a distance. Television, teleconferencing, telemarketing, telecommuting, telecommunications.

telemedicine
Doing medical activities (consultation, taking part in a conference, teaching) at a distance using communications technology.

telnet
Protocol on the Internet that allows you to log on to a distant computer and run programs. Many computer databases are open to the public via telnet.

template
Preset format, such as for a publication.

terabyte
One trillion bytes, abbreviated as TB.

terminal
Point in a mainframe system where the monitor and keyboard are located. Terminal emulation refers to the kind of keyboard a mainframe expects to see.

text box
Blank rectangular area on a computer screen where you type in text. On the Web, text boxes are used in forms to collect information.

text-to-speech
Computer program that reads text aloud.

thesaurus
Book or program with synonyms.

thinko
Transient error in brain function, often transmitted to the fingers as a typo.

thread
Series of messages on a newsgroup about a particular topic. When anyone answers another person's message, that starts a thread.

thumbnail
Small version of a picture which when clicked often brings up the larger picture.

toolbar
Group of buttons on a program or Web site. Each button activates one function.

trash
Temporary holding area for deleted files or messages. You can retrieve items from the trash until you empty it.

Tron
1982 movie about virtual reality.

truncation
Using a wild card character to search for a broad range of words. The asterisk (*) is often used as a wild card. For example, typing hep* will find heparin, hepatitis, hepatic.

turbo nerd
High-powered geek.

tutorial
Step-by-step instructions for a procedure. Sometimes loosely used for any handout or information.

U

UMLS
Unified Medical Language System. System for finding information located in different computer systems using different terminologies, concepts, and formats. Can link databases, patient records, bibliographic citations, expert systems. The NLM UMLS includes a metathesaurus, Lexicon, Semantic Network, and Information Sources Map.

UNIX
Common operating system used on Internet host computers.

update
1. To enter new or changed information.
2. On MEDLINE a function whereby you can set up an automatic weekly search. Limited to certain institutions.

upgrade
To install new hardware or software.

upload
To transfer files from your desktop computer to a distant computer.

URL
Uniform Resource Locator. Address of a Web site.

Usenet
General name for the whole collection of newsgroups on the Internet.

V

virtual
Simulated, not real. A picture of a tomato is virtual: you can't eat it.

virtual reality
Three-dimensional images on a computer created with VRML.

virus
Small program created to deliberately and covertly lodge itself in a computer, often doing damage to the files or programs.

voice mail
Ability of a telephone to have mailboxes where people can call in to leave messages. Voice mail is similar to an answering machine, but has many more functions.

VRML
Virtual Reality Markup Language. Protocol for displaying three-dimensional images on a computer which you can enter, go behind, etc.

W

WAIS (Wide Area Information Server)
Method of indexing documents that preceded Web search engines.

WAN
Wide Area Network. A network that spans an area larger than a single building. See LAN.

Web
Abbreviation for the World Wide Web. Also written as WWW or W3.

wedgitude
Between a rock and a hard place.

weighted search
Giving more emphasis (weight) to a word when using a search engine.

wellness
Emphasizing a better state of health rather than prevention or cure of disease.

wide area network
Physical network that can span several miles. See *local area network*.

whiteboard
Whiteboard programs allow several people to see a "space" with written comments, a spreadsheet, or pictures.

wild card character
Character which stands for any other typed character when doing a search. See *truncation*.

window
Rectangular area on the screen which shows a program or part of a program. You can change the size or shape of a window with the mouse.

Windows
An operating system that coordinates the parts of a computer such as the keyboard, mouse, monitor, hard drive, CD-ROM. Different versions are called Windows 3.1, Windows 95, Windows 97, Windows NT.

winsock
Software that Windows computers use to set up a TCP/IP connection.

wizard
Programmed, step-by-step process of accomplishing a task. When you start a wizard, you are given a series of windows with choices for each step.

word processor
Program for typing; also called text editor.

word wrapping
Function that automatically brings the word to the next line in a word processor.

workstation
Personal computer which is connected to a network, allowing it to exchange files and information.

World Wide Web
All the computers and documents on the Internet that are linked together using Hypertext Transport Protocol (HTTP). Also written as Web, WWW, or W3.

worm
Program that propagates itself as it travels. See *Internet Worm, the Great.*

Z

Zip drive
Drive with removable disks similar to a floppy, each of which can hold 100 megabytes. For backup or transfer of large files.

F Index

The index does not include names of the approximately 750 Web sites listed in this book. If you want to find a Web site, look in the chapter devoted to that topic. If you already know the name of a Web site ("Oncolink"), you can use one of the major search engines to find it.

A

B

C

D

E

F

G

H

N

O

P

Q

R

S

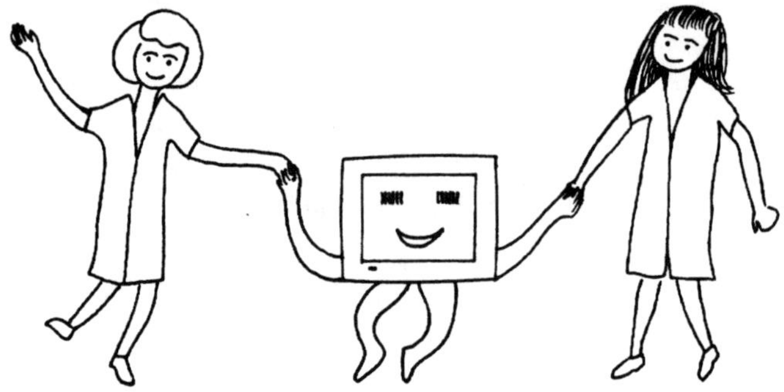

Order Form

A Pocket Guide to the Medical Internet (ISBN 0-9651412-3-3)
The Internet Workbook for Health Professionals (ISBN 0-9651412-4-1)

See our Web site for distributors and bookstores:

http://NewWindPub.com

You can order directly from New Wind. Books are shipped next day.

Please send ___ copies of the Workbook @ $19.95 each $________
___ copies of the Pocket Guide @ $7.95 each $________

Shipping:

Workbook	$3.00 ($1.00 extra copies.)	Foreign:	$7.00	($2.00 extra copies)
Pocket	$1.00 ($0.50 extra copies)	Foreign:	$2.00	($1.00 extra copies)

Shipping: $________

Tax: (California residents only)
Workbook $1.55 each
Pocket Guide $0.62 each **Tax:** $________

TOTAL ENCLOSED: $________

Your name: ______________________
Address: ______________________
____
____

Email address: ______________________

Send check or money order to:

NEW WIND PUBLISHING
BOX 161613
SACRAMENTO, CA 95816-1613

Visa and MasterCard accepted

Card number: ______________________
Expiration Date: ______________________

Questions? Call or fax: (916) 451-9039
Email: info@NewWindPub.com

(Links available at http://NewWindPub.com/workbook)

G Quick Reference

DIRECTORIES OF MEDICAL SITES

Medical Matrix	http://www.medmatrix.org
MedWeb	http://www.cc.emory.edu/whscl/medweb.html
Hardin	http://www.arcade.uiowa.edu/hardin-www/md.html

SEARCH ENGINES

AtoZ	http://www.HealthAtoZ.com
Medical World	http://pride-sun.poly.edu
Health On The Net	http://www.hon.ch
Medis	http://www.docnet.org.uk/medisn/searchs.html
AltaVista	http://www.altavista.digital.com

MEDICATIONS

Rx List	http://www.rxlist.com
Gold Multimedia Database	http://www.cponline.gsm.com

CONSUMER INFORMATION FOR THE PUBLIC

Healthfinder	http://www.healthfinder.gov
MedHelp	http://medhlp.netusa.net
Healthtouch	http://www.healthtouch.com
HealthAnswers	http://www.healthanswers.com

JOURNALS

Elec. Journals	http://www.hslib.washington.edu/journals
Kansas Univ.	http://www.kumc.edu/dykes/journals/display.html

MEDLINE LITERATURE SEARCH

Natl. Lib. of Medicine	http://www.ncbi.nlm.nih.gov/PubMed
Medical Matrix	http://www.medmatrix.org/SPages/Medline.stm

TESTS AND PROCEDURES

HealthAnswers	http://www.healthanswers.com (click Search; (any topic); Tests; Tests and Procedures).
Health Gate	http://www.healthgate.com